This unique cookbook is provided as a service of Hoechst Canada Inc., the makers of…

Diaßeta®

(Glyburide)

Commitment to research and patient education in the field of diabetes has always been one of our major goals.

Your commitment on the insistance of brand name pharmaceutical products helps immensely in the achievement of these goals.

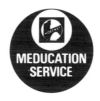

MEDUCATION SERVICE

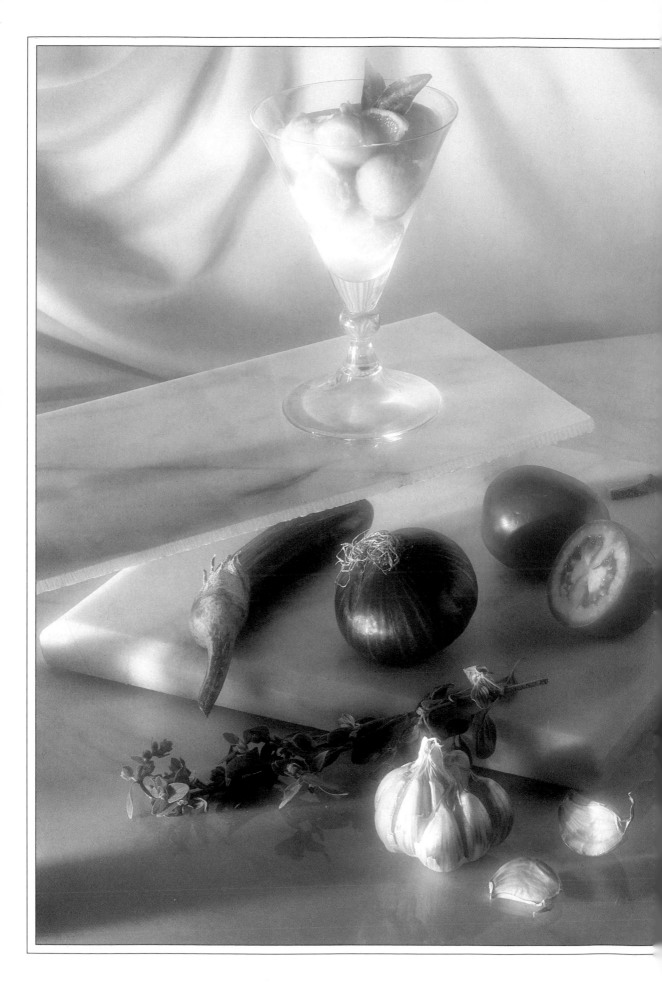

RECIPES FOR GOOD HEALTH

NEW
DIABETIC
COOKERY

Written and compiled by

Barbara Davidson, SRD

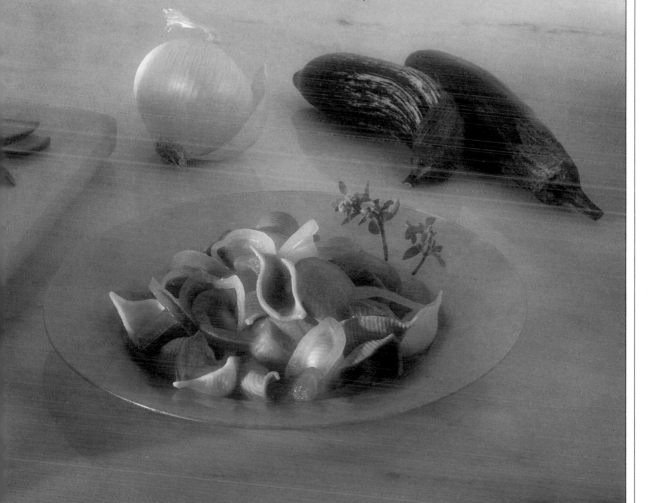

OCTOPUS BOOKS

ACKNOWLEDGMENTS

The publisher acknowledges the following photographers: Bryce Attwell pages 28–9, Rex Bamber pages 49, 52, 56–7, 67, 70–1, 74; Robert Golden pages 38, 47; Melvin Grey pages 20, 112; Gina Harris page 93; Roger Phillips pages 10–11, 42; Clive Streeter page 108; Grant Symon cover, pages 2–3, 61, 88–9, 100–1, 103–4, 118–19, 122; Paul Williams page 92. Other photographs were supplied by: American Rice Council pages 35, 79; American Spice Trade Association page 15; Apple and Pear Development Council page 25; Campbell Soup Company page 97; Carmel Produce Information Bureau page 35; Hellmans page 32; Sea Fish Kitchen page 84. Cookware, dishes and cutlery used in Grant Symon's photographs were provided by: Elizabeth David, 46 Bourne Street, London SW1; Fieldhouse, 89 Wandsworth Bridge Road, London SW6; Graham and Green, 4 and 7 Elgin Crescent, London W11; David Mellor, 4 Sloane Square, London SW1, 26 James Street, Covent Garden, London WC2, and 66 King Street, Manchester, M2; Smash and Grab, 662 Fulham Road, London SW6.

Cover illustration: Peach and raspberry cheesecake, page 75; Spiced chicken, page 88. Title spread illustration: Orange sorbet, page 68; Pasta with ratatouille sauce, page 61.

The energy and fibre values included in the recipes were based in part on information from *The Composition of Foods* by R.A. McCance and E.M. Widdowson, 4th revised edition, HMSO 1978, by A.A. Paul and D.A.T. Southgate.

COOKING NOTE

The measurements in the recipes are given in both metric and imperial units. Use whichever system you are familiar with, but do not mix the two as the equivalents are not exact.

When spoonfuls are mentioned use level spoons:
1 teaspoon = 5 ml.
1 tablespoon = 15 ml.
Australian readers who use a 20 ml tablespoon should use 3×5 ml teaspoons to get the correct measure for the recipes in this book.

This edition first published 1986 by
Octopus Books Ltd
59 Grosvenor Street, London W1

© 1986 Octopus Books Ltd

Reprinted 1988, 1990

ISBN 0 7064 2624 X

Phototypeset by Tradespools Ltd
Frome, Somerset, England

Produced by Mandarin Offset
Printed and bound in Hong Kong

CONTENTS

HEALTHY EATING FOR DIABETICS

Since 1982, there has been something of a revolution in the advice given to diabetics about their diet. Before then, a book such as this would not have been feasible. The 'rules' about what was and was not suitable for diabetic people were so strict that the idea of a cookery book that could be used by diabetics and their families and friends would have been out of the question.

This, however, *is* such a book, full of interesting and nutritious recipes that can be slotted into the diet of any member of the family. The recipes cover all meals and include ideas for quick dishes and some specifically aimed at children.

But before making any changes to your diet you should consult your doctor or dietitian. You can then be sure that your diet continues to agree with any other diabetic treatment you may be prescribed.

THE TRADITIONAL DIABETIC DIET

Some people who suffer from diabetes can control the level of sugar in their blood by dietary control alone, whereas others need help from tablets or injections of insulin.

In the past, diets for both insulin-dependent and non-insulin dependent diabetics allowed restricted amounts of carbohydrate – both starchy food and refined sugars. It was thought that any excess carbohydrate, especially refined sugars, above the amount required for normal activity would immediately cause the level of blood sugar to rise and therefore cause problems such as hyperglycaemia.

While so much attention was paid to the amount of carbohydrate in the diabetic diet, there was little or no concern about the proportion of fat or protein eaten, and the dietary fibre content was never even taken into consideration. The total energy content of the diet – expressed as calories (kcal) or joules (kJ) – was only thought important for diabetics who were overweight and needed to follow a weight-reducing diet to achieve better control over their blood sugar levels.

Many diabetics have lived for years following such a diet, and have achieved good diabetic control. However, it was very restrictive and often unappetizing. It also took little account of individual variation in activity or lifestyle and was hard to fit in with family meals. In addition, these traditional diets were particularly difficult to manage when on holiday or entertaining or when cooking for young children, and they set diabetics apart and made them feel and be treated as 'different'.

NEW RESEARCH

For the past 60 years or so, doctors have been investigating the effect of various types of carbohydrates on blood sugar levels. Part of this research focused on diabetes in different ethnic groups. For example, it was found that the incidence of diabetes increased dramatically when certain tribes of American Indians changed from their traditional diet, which was very rich in fibre and contained a high proportion of vegetables, to a more 'Western' diet – that is, one containing a greater proportion of refined foods, such as white flour, sugar and white rice, and convenience foods in general.

Further research revealed that, when foods rich in both fibre and unrefined carbohydrate were eaten, the sugar levels in the blood did not rise as high or as quickly as might have been predicted. Also, the type of fibre in beans, pulses and oats was found to have a protective effect on the release of sugars from foods, slowing it down so that any insulin injected into or produced by the body had a better chance of controlling blood sugar levels effectively. Fibre helps keep cholesterol levels down, too.

High-fibre, high-carbohydrate foods have the added advantage of being low in fat. This has to be good news for diabetics, in whom uncontrolled weight can mean uncontrolled diabetes. Research into heart disease – from which diabetics are slightly more at risk – has implicated fat as a major contributory factor, and particularly saturated (mainly animal) fat, found in butter, cheese, red meat and so on. It is a very good idea to cut down on this, and change to moderate amounts of polyunsaturated (primarily vegetable) fats and oils.

THE NEW DIABETIC DIET

CHANGING TO HIGH-FIBRE CARBOHYDRATE FOODS

In essence, the new diabetic diet is one that concentrates on the total number of calories to be eaten every day to suit a person's height and build. Fibre-rich foods should be used as carbohydrate sources to provide nutritious filling meals that will help keep blood sugar and blood fat levels low. The best high-carbohydrate foods are:
- Pulses such as lentils, kidney beans, haricot beans, and so on.
- Whole-grain cereals such as wholemeal flour, bread and pasta and brown rice.
- Vegetables such as jacket potatoes.
- Fresh fruits, which have a natural fibre content, especially those, such as apples and pears, that can be eaten unpeeled.

As can be seen from the table below, the amounts of carbohydrate recommended in the new diet are substantially greater than those in the traditional diet for the same number of calories/joules.

To help you achieve these target amounts of carbohydrate, the recipes in this book include analyses of carbohydrate (CHO) content per portion in grams and units, energy content in kcal and kJ.

It is important to remember that although the sugars are also carbohydrates, the type you should be eating is *high-fibre* carbohydrate, which will be absorbed slowly in the body and does not result in a sudden rise in blood sugar levels.

Calories/joules per day (as advised by dietitian/doctor)	TRADITIONAL DIET Grams/units carbohydrate per day	NEW DIET Grams/units carbohydrate per day
1000 kcal/4200 kJ	100 g/10 units	140 g/14 units
1500 kcal/6300 kJ	150 g/15 units	210 g/21 units
2000 kcal/8400 kJ	200 g/20 units	280 g/28 units
2500 kcal/10,500 kJ	250 g/25 units	340 g/34 units

TIMING YOUR MEALS

If your diet is controlled by insulin, it is important to plan your mealtimes according to the insulin you are taking, and to spread the carbohydrate in your diet evenly throughout the day.

If, on the other hand, your diet is controlled by tablets or by diet alone, then it is also sensible to have regular meals and to ensure that a larger proportion of the foods you eat is high-fibre carbohydrate, to keep blood sugar as even as possible.

In every case, you should take the advice of your doctor and dietitian concerning all aspects of your diet. You should particularly avoid prolonged gaps without food.

Although it is important to have the carbohydrate in your diet evenly distributed throughout the day, the fat and protein content of the diet can be more flexible. Therefore a meal with a higher protein or fat content than usual – perhaps for a celebration – can be balanced by lighter meals during the rest of the day.

If you find yourself missing a meal, a wholemeal bread sandwich would make a satisfying snack. In addition, your body will need extra energy when you take part in sports or perform any other vigorous activity, and this is best provided by taking some extra carbohydrate beforehand. One of the recipes in the baking section may be useful here.

WATCHING YOUR WEIGHT

Everyone, diabetic or not, should avoid becoming overweight. Keeping an eye on the total number of calories in your daily diet helps you to do this.

If you are overweight and your doctor recommends that your diabetes can be controlled by diet alone, you can do this by carefully controlling your daily energy intake and losing any excess weight.

If you have been prescribed tablets or insulin for your diabetes, you should still try to maintain the correct weight for your height, build and age by controlling how much high-energy food you eat. This is because excessive weight leads to a loss of sensitivity to insulin. Happily, once excess weight is lost, you body's insulin sensitivity will be restored.

Fat and protein, as well as carbohydrate, all provide energy in the form of calories/joules; but fat contains more than twice the energy, gram for gram, of protein and carbohydrate. If you find your weight creeping up, the easiest way to decrease your energy intake is to cut down on the amount of fat you eat by altering the types of food in your diet or the way they are cooked.(See 'Cooking hints' opposite.) You can eat more low-fat foods such as skimmed milk, cottage cheese, poultry and fish, and avoid the red meats that contain relatively large amounts of 'invisible' fat.

Refined sugar, although a carbohydrate, is absorbed very rapidly into the bloodstream and can play havoc with diabetic control; in addition, eating sugar leads to weight gain. It has no nutritional value, merely providing what are known as 'empty calories', and should be omitted from your diet. Watch out for proprietary diabetic foods: these contain fructose or sorbitol instead of glucose, but have the same amount of calories.

You should, of course, still carry an emergency supply of sugar with you in case your blood sugar unexpectedly drops too low (hypoglycaemic attack). As you will see in this book, most recipes can be adapted to avoid sugar, and much tastier results are often achieved. If a sweet taste is desired, use an artificial sweetener or, even better, add dried fruits to a recipe.

EATING OUT

The advice in this book, as well as the recipes, should give you some idea of which meals to try when eating out. The best thing to do is avoid deeply fried foods, and those that are covered in heavy sauces that disguise not only what lies beneath but also the ingredients of the sauce itself. Most restaurants will offer a choice of vegetables, allowing you to choose, for example, a jacket potato in preference to fried potatoes, or a crisp fruit salad rather than a heavy pastry-and-cream concoction.

SHOPPING

Most ingredients found in the following chapters are easily available, although one or two items from the recipes in the international section might necessitate an exploratory trip to specialist food shops less frequently visited.

Long-grain brown rice, wholemeal flour and wholemeal pasta can be found on most supermarket shelves today. If they are not, try a health food shop, of which there is now a growing number.

COOKING HINTS

- Grilling, boiling, poaching or steaming foods instead of frying them can result in tastier, healthier meals.
- If using an artificial sweetener, add it towards the end of a recipe (if not mentioned in the method) to avoid any bitter aftertaste.
- Plain, unsweetened yogurt can be used in place of cream and soured cream in recipes or as a topping—on jacket potatoes or fruit salad, for example.
- Natural bran can be added to dishes to provide extra fibre without adding to the carbohydrate or calorie/joule content. However, don't be heavyhanded with it, as only small amounts (around 2 teaspoons a day) will speed up the action of the large intestine.
- Pressure cooking is a good method of cooking vegetables, as it conserves taste without losing mineral and vitamin content.

- Different types of lentils and pulses require different soaking/cooking times, so follow the advice given in each recipe or provided on the packet.
- You can use skimmed or semi-skimmed milk – which contains little or no fat but retains the protein, minerals and vitamins – in place of whole milk without altering the carbohydrate content. Comparative energy values are:
    100 ml/4 fl oz whole milk =
    65 kcal/270 kJ
    100 ml/4 fl oz semi-skimmed milk =
    50 kcal/205 kJ
    100 ml/4 fl oz skimmed milk =
    35 kcal/140 kJ
- When using an alcoholic drink in a cooked dish, the alcohol in it evaporates, leaving behind only the flavour. Therefore there is no need to worry about the effects of alcohol on your condition when it is used in cooking.

USING THE ANALYSES

In each recipe in this book, you will find a list setting out the total energy – expressed as calories (kcal) and joules (kJ) – in each serving as well as the amounts in grams (and, in the case of carbohydrate, 10-gram units) of carbohydrate (CHO), fibre, fat and protein.

Your doctor or dietitian will be able to guide you towards the right energy level for your weight and height. Your daily energy intake will dictate the amount of carbohydrate you need. You should also aim for at least 30 g of fibre each day, and no more than 35 per cent of your daily calorie intake should be made up of fat. The amount of protein you need will depend on your age, height and build; for

adults, it will vary between 55 and 90 g per day, depending on these factors.

To help with the mental arithmetic, you will find some examples of daily meal plans at various energy levels, with the corresponding amounts of carbohydrate, at the end of this book.

It is generally agreed that a high-carbohydrate, high-fibre, low-fat diet is the most beneficial for diabetics. The recipes in *New Diabetic Cookery* can help you achieve this, as well as improving the nutrition of the entire family.

Breakfast Recipes

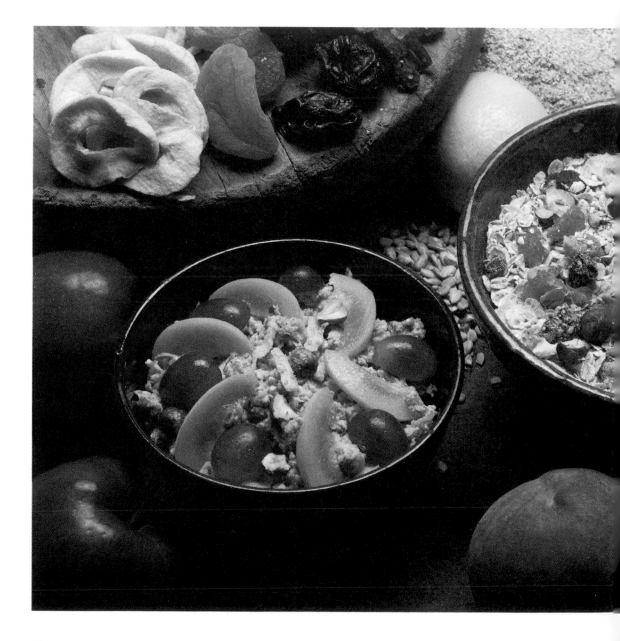

STORECUPBOARD MUESLI

225 g/8 oz rolled oats
100 g/4 oz Bran Flakes cereal
50 g/2 oz chopped nuts
50 g/2 oz seedless raisins and coarsely chopped
*   dried fruit*

MAKES about 450 g/1 lb
Total recipe:
Energy 1550 kcal/6520 kJ
CHO 250 g (25 units)
Fibre 47 g **Fat** 47 g **Protein** 46 g

Place the rolled oats in a sieve and shake vigorously to remove the 'flour'. Combine the oats in a mixing bowl with the other ingredients. Store in an air-tight container and serve at breakfast with a little chopped fresh fruit and some plain unsweetened yogurt.

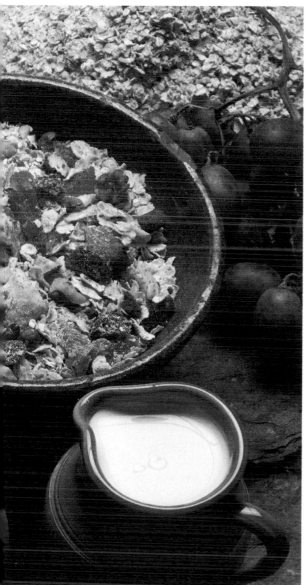

SWISS BREAKFAST

1 tablespoon wheatgerm
1 tablespoon rolled oats
4 tablespoons water
1 teaspoon lemon juice
1 dessert apple, unpeeled and coarsely grated
2 tablespoons plain unsweetened yogurt
25 g/1 oz hazelnuts, chopped

SERVES 1
Per serving:
Energy 300 kcal/1250 kJ
CHO 31 g (3 units)
Fibre 11 g **Fat** 14 g **Protein** 12 g

Put the wheatgerm, oats and water in a serving bowl. Cover and leave in the refrigerator overnight.

Then combine the oat mixture with the lemon juice, grated apple and yogurt. Sprinkle on the nuts and serve immediately, with fresh fruit in season.

LEFT: SWISS BREAKFAST; RIGHT: STORE–CUPBOARD MUESLI

YOGURT AND OAT MUESLI

250 ml / 8 fl oz plain unsweetened yogurt
75 g / 3 oz rolled oats
4 tablespoons raisins
2 dessert apples, unpeeled and coarsely grated
4 tablespoons chopped walnuts
2 tablespoons lemon juice

SERVES 2
Per serving:
Energy 210 kcal / 900 kJ
CHO 30 g (3 units)
Fibre 3 g   **Fat** 1 g   **Protein** 4 g

Put the yogurt into a large mixing bowl and add the remaining ingredients. Mix thoroughly and leave to stand for a few hours, or refrigerate overnight before serving.

ORANGE AND PRUNE CRUNCH

175 ml / 6 fl oz plain unsweetened yogurt
¼ teaspoon ground ginger
2 large oranges, peel, pith and membrane
    removed
75 g / 3 oz cooked prunes, chopped
50 g / 2 oz rolled oats

SERVES 4
Per serving:
Energy 110 kcal / 460 kJ
CHO 20 g (2 units)
Fibre 3 g   **Fat** 1 g   **Protein** 4 g

Combine the yogurt and the ginger. Slice the orange flesh thinly. Mix with the yogurt, chopped prunes and oats. Spoon into individual dishes and serve.

PRUNE WHIP

200 g / 7 oz prunes, soaked overnight in cold
    water
1 tablespoon powdered gelatine
4 tablespoons water
450 ml / ¾ pint plain unsweetened yogurt
1 teaspoon lemon juice
TO DECORATE
25 g / 1 oz walnuts, chopped

SERVES 4
Per serving:
Energy 130 kcal / 550 kJ
CHO 15 g (1.5 units)
Fibre 4 g   **Fat** 4 g   **Protein** 7 g

Put the prunes and soaking liquid into a saucepan and simmer until soft. Purée in a blender with a little of the juice.

Soak the gelatine in the water in a heatproof bowl, then place over a pan of gently simmering water until dissolved. When cool, add to the prunes with the yogurt and lemon juice.

Spoon into glasses and leave to set. Decorate with the chopped nuts.

BREAKFAST SCRAMBLE

15 g / ½ oz polyunsaturated margarine
3 green peppers, cored, seeded and chopped
4 eggs
75 ml / 3 fl oz skimmed milk
50 g / 2 oz ham, chopped
4 slices wholemeal bread, toasted
50 g / 2 oz Edam cheese, grated

SERVES 4
Per serving:
Energy 225 kcal / 935 kJ
CHO 15 g (1.5 units)
Fibre 2 g **Fat** 10 g **Protein** 15 g

Melt the margarine in a non-stick pan and cook the green peppers gently. Beat the eggs and milk, pour over the peppers and cook in the usual way. When almost cooked add the chopped ham. Serve on slices of toast sprinkled with the grated cheese.

BROWN RICE PIPÉRADE

1 tablespoon polyunsaturated vegetable oil
1 large onion, chopped
2 carrots, scrubbed and diced
450 g / 1 lb spinach, shredded
1 tablespoon chopped parsley
225 g / 8 oz brown rice, cooked
salt and freshly ground black pepper
3 eggs, beaten
½ teaspoon Worcestershire sauce

SERVES 4
Per serving:
Energy 205 kcal / 860 kJ
CHO 50 g (5 units)
Fibre 4 g **Fat** 9 g **Protein** 13 g

Heat the oil in a large frying pan. Add the onion, carrots and spinach. Stir-fry until the onions are translucent and carrots and spinach tender. Add the parsley, rice, salt and pepper to the vegetables. Add the eggs and Worcestershire sauce. Stir the mixture until the eggs have set.

Serve the dish immediately.

Soups
& Starters

SPICED VEGETABLE SOUP

1 litre/1¾ pints beef stock
1 litre/1¾ pints water
1 × 250 ml (8 fl oz) can tomato juice
2 tablespoons finely chopped onion
1¼ teaspoons crushed thyme leaves
1 garlic clove, crushed
1 teaspoon salt
225 g/8 oz chuck steak, cut into 1 cm/½ inch
  cubes
½ teaspoon whole black peppercorns
4 whole cloves

225 g/8 oz potatoes, peeled and cut into 1 cm/
  ½ inch cubes
100 g/4 oz marrow or courgettes, peeled and cut
  into 1 cm/½ inch cubes
275 g/10 oz cabbage, coarsely sliced
100 g/4 oz carrots, scrubbed and sliced
100 g/4 oz celery, sliced
2 corn-on-the-cobs (about 350 g/12 oz), cut into
  2.5 cm/1 inch lengths
TO GARNISH
chopped parsley

SERVES 6–8

6 servings
Per serving:

Energy 200 kcal/820 kJ		
CHO 25 g (2.5 units)		
Fibre 5 g	**Fat** 6 g	**Protein** 11 g

8 servings
Per serving:

Energy 150 kcal/615 kJ		
CHO 20 g (2 units)		
Fibre 3 g	**Fat** 4 g	**Protein** 8 g

Place the beef stock, water, tomato juice, onion, thyme, garlic, salt and meat in a pan. Add the black peppercorns and cloves, tied in muslin if liked. Bring to the boil, cover and simmer for 40 minutes.

Add the potatoes and marrow or courgettes. Cover and simmer for 10 minutes. Add the cabbage, carrots, celery and corn. Cover and simmer for about 10 minutes or until the meat and vegetables are tender. Serve the soup sprinkled with chopped parsley.

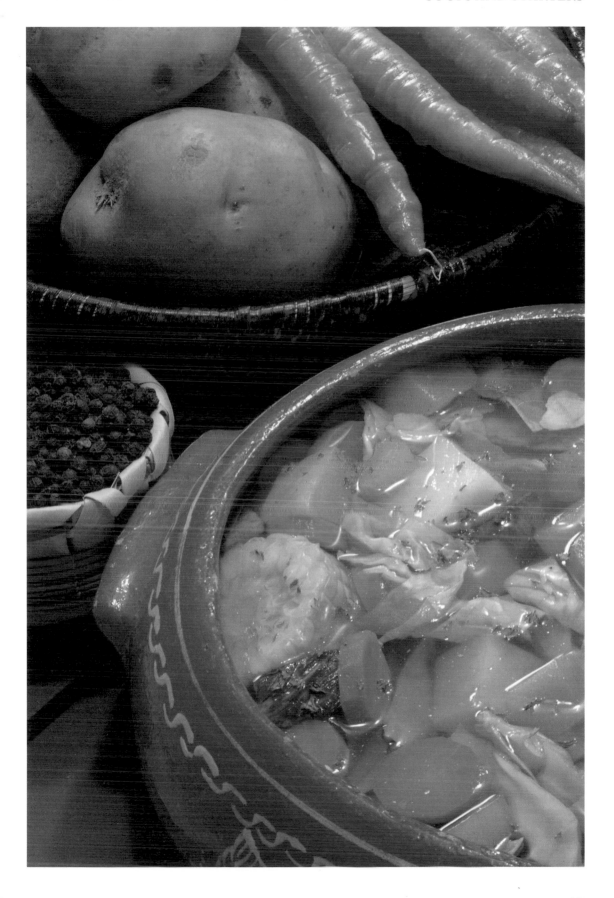

VEGETABLE SOUP

25 g/1 oz polyunsaturated margarine
1 leek, cut into 1 cm/½ inch pieces
1 celery stick, chopped
1 large potato, peeled and sliced
1 carrot, scraped and grated
300 ml/½ pint chicken stock
150 ml/¼ pint dry cider
salt
freshly ground black pepper

SERVES 2
Per serving:
Energy 180 kcal/750 kJ
CHO 14 g (1.5 units)
Fibre 3 g   **Fat** 10 g   **Protein** 3 g

Melt the margarine in a saucepan and add the leek. Cover and cook gently for 1 minute.

Add the celery and potato and cook gently for 5 minutes. Add the carrot, stock, cider and salt and pepper to taste. Bring to the boil, cover and simmer for 40 minutes until all the vegetables are tender. Adjust the seasoning and serve hot with grated cheese and wholemeal bread.

ICED WATERCRESS AND LEMON SOUP

2 bunches watercress, washed and excess stalks
    removed
1 onion, finely chopped
450 ml/¾ pint chicken stock
300 ml/½ pint skimmed milk
2 tablespoons finely grated lemon rind
salt
freshly ground black pepper
150 ml/¼ pint plain unsweetened yogurt

SERVES 4
Per serving:
Energy 40 kcal/180 kJ
CHO 5 g (0.5 units)
Fibre 0 g   **Fat** 0 g   **Protein** 4 g

Chop the watercress leaves roughly (re-serving a few of the best sprigs for garnish) and put into a pan with the onion, stock, milk, lemon rind, salt and pepper to taste. Simmer gently for 30 minutes. Purée in a blender or rub through a fine sieve and allow to cool.

Stir in the yogurt, adjust the seasoning and chill. Serve topped with small sprigs of fresh watercress.

CARROT AND TURNIP SOUP

15 g/½ oz polyunsaturated margarine
225 g/8 oz carrots, scraped and sliced
225 g/8 oz turnips, peeled and sliced
1 litre/1¾ pints chicken stock
salt
freshly ground black pepper
2 teaspoons ground coriander
1 teaspoon ground cumin
1 tablespoon finely chopped coriander leaves

SERVES 4
Per serving:
Energy 45 kcal/190 kJ
CHO 5 g (0.5 units)
Fibre 2 g   **Fat** 3 g   **Protein** 0 g

Heat the margarine in a saucepan, add the carrots and turnips and cook gently for about 6 minutes, stirring occasionally. Heat the stock in a separate saucepan and pour it over the vegetables. Bring to the boil, add salt and pepper, and simmer for 30 minutes, covered. Put through a coarse food mill or blender and return to the clean pan. Reheat, adding more salt and pepper as needed. Add the spices and the chopped coriander leaves, mix well, and stand for 5 minutes before serving.

GREEN GARDEN SOUP

4 celery sticks, chopped
2 leeks, washed and shredded
1 bunch watercress stalks, trimmed
3 courgettes, thinly sliced
600 ml / 1 pint chicken stock
salt
freshly ground black pepper
1 garlic clove, crushed
small bunch of parsley

150 ml / ¼ pint plain unsweetened yogurt
TO GARNISH
chopped fresh chives

SERVES 4
Per serving:
Energy 40 kcal/155 kJ
CHO 0 g (0 units)
Fibre 1 g **Fat** 0 g **Protein** 4 g

Put the celery, leeks, watercress and courgettes into a saucepan together with the chicken stock, salt and pepper to taste, garlic and parsley. Simmer gently until the vegetables are just tender – about 15 minutes.

Purée in a blender or food processor until smooth. Cool, then stir in half the yogurt. Chill.

Serve in soup bowls with a little of the remaining yogurt swirled on top of each portion. Garnish with chopped chives.

GARDENERS' BROTH

25 g / 1 oz polyunsaturated margarine
1 rasher lean bacon, rinded and diced
2–3 small onions, sliced
2–3 small carrots, scrubbed and sliced
small piece of turnip
1 litre / 1¾ pints stock or water
2 tomatoes, skinned and sliced
2–3 runner beans, topped and tailed
few young cabbage leaves
salt
freshly ground black pepper

pinch of mixed herbs
25 g / 1 oz wholemeal macaroni
TO GARNISH
grated cheese
1 tablespoon finely chopped parsley

SERVES 4
Per serving:
Energy 120 kcal/500 kJ
CHO 10 g (1 unit)
Fibre 2 g **Fat** 8 g **Protein** 3 g

Melt the margarine in a saucepan, add the bacon and onions and cook until soft. Add the carrots and turnip and cook for a further 5 minutes. Pour in the stock or water and bring to the boil. Add the remaining vegetables, salt, pepper and herbs, then cover and simmer for 45 minutes. Add the macaroni and simmer for a further 15 minutes. Serve piping hot, sprinkled with grated cheese and chopped fresh parsley.

PURÉE OF CELERY SOUP

50 g/2 oz polyunsaturated margarine
450 g/1 lb celery, cut into 1 cm/½ inch pieces
225 g/8 oz potatoes, peeled and cut into 2.5 cm/
    1 inch cubes
1.2 litres/2 pints chicken stock or water
1 bouquet garni

salt
freshly ground black pepper
120 ml/4 fl oz skimmed milk
TO GARNISH
chopped parsley

SERVES 4–6
4 servings
Per serving:
Energy 170 kcal/700 kJ
CHO 15 g (1.5 units)
Fibre 3 g **Fat** 11 g **Protein** 3 g

6 servings
Per serving:
Energy 100 kcal/430 kJ
CHO 10 g (1 unit)
Fibre 2 g **Fat** 6 g **Protein** 2 g

Heat the margarine in a large pan, toss the vegetables in this. Add the stock or water, bouquet garni, salt and pepper. Simmer for 30 minutes.

Remove the herbs if desired, although these can be puréed with the other ingredients. Sieve, or purée the mixture in a blender or food processor. Return the soup to the pan with the milk and heat. Garnish with the parsley.

LENTIL SOUP WITH COCONUT

1 tablespoon polyunsaturated vegetable oil
1 onion, chopped
1–2 garlic cloves, chopped
1½ teaspoons cumin seeds or ground cumin
4 cardamoms or ¼ teaspoon ground cardamom
1 carrot, scraped and chopped
1 teaspoon ground turmeric
175 g/6 oz red lentils, rinsed thoroughly
1.5 litres/2½ pints chicken stock
2 bay leaves
1 teaspoon ground coriander

salt
freshly ground black pepper
40 g/1½ oz creamed coconut, cut into small
    pieces
1 tablespoon tomato purée

SERVES 4
Per serving:
Energy 195 kcal/830 kJ
CHO 25 g (2.5 units)
Fibre 5 g **Fat** 6 g **Protein** 11 g

Heat the oil in a large, deep saucepan, add the onion and garlic and cook for 2 minutes. If using whole spices, crush the cumin seeds and cardamoms together with the back of a spoon in a cup, or use a pestle and mortar. Discard the cardamom husks. Add the crushed or ground cumin and cardamom to the onion and garlic with the carrot and turmeric, and cook for 2 minutes.

Add the lentils, discarding any discoloured ones, stock, bay leaves and coriander. Bring to the boil slowly, then add salt and pepper. Cover and simmer for 45–60 minutes or until the lentils are soft. Add the creamed coconut and stir until melted. Stir in the tomato purée. Remove the bay leaves and purée the soup in a blender. Return the soup to the rinsed pan and reheat gently. Taste and adjust the seasoning and serve very hot.

HEARTY FISH SOUP

350 g/12 oz potatoes, washed and sliced
300 ml/½ pint skimmed milk
300 ml/½ pint water
salt and freshly ground black pepper
350 g/12 oz whiting fillets, skinned and cut into
    2 cm/¾ inch cubes

4 tablespoons peas
4 tablespoons sweetcorn
2 tablespoons tomato purée
lemon juice

SERVES 2–4

2 servings			**4 servings**		
Per serving:			**Per serving:**		
Energy 420 kcal/1790 kJ			**Energy** 190 kcal/805 kJ		
CHO 50 g (5 units)			**CHO** 25 g (2.5 units)		
Fibre 8 g	**Fat** 5 g	**Protein** 41 g	**Fibre** 4 g	**Fat** 1 g	**Protein** 20 g

Place the potatoes, milk, water, and salt and pepper in a saucepan and simmer gently for 10 minutes. Add the fish with the peas and sweetcorn. Simmer, covered, for a further 10–15 minutes. Just before serving, stir in the tomato purée and lemon juice to taste and serve hot.

SPICY LENTIL SOUP

450 g/1 lb red lentils, rinsed thoroughly
25 g/1 oz polyunsaturated margarine
2 medium onions, chopped
2 garlic cloves, chopped
2 celery sticks, chopped
1 × 400 g (14 oz) can tomatoes
1 chilli, seeded and chopped (optional)
1 teaspoon paprika
1 teaspoon chilli powder
1 teaspoon ground cumin

1 teaspoon salt
freshly ground black pepper
1.2 litres/2 pints chicken stock or water

SERVES 8

Per serving:		
Energy 205 kcal/875 kJ		
CHO 32 g (3 units)		
Fibre 7 g	**Fat** 3 g	**Protein** 14 g

Discard any discoloured lentils. Melt the margarine in a large saucepan over a low heat and cook the onions, garlic and celery until soft. Add the lentils to the vegetables with the tomatoes. Stir well to combine. Add the remaining ingredients, cover and simmer gently for about 2 hours. Add a little more water if the soup becomes too thick and take care not to let the mixture burn on the bottom of the saucepan.

Serve hot with wholemeal toast. *Illustrated on page 20.*

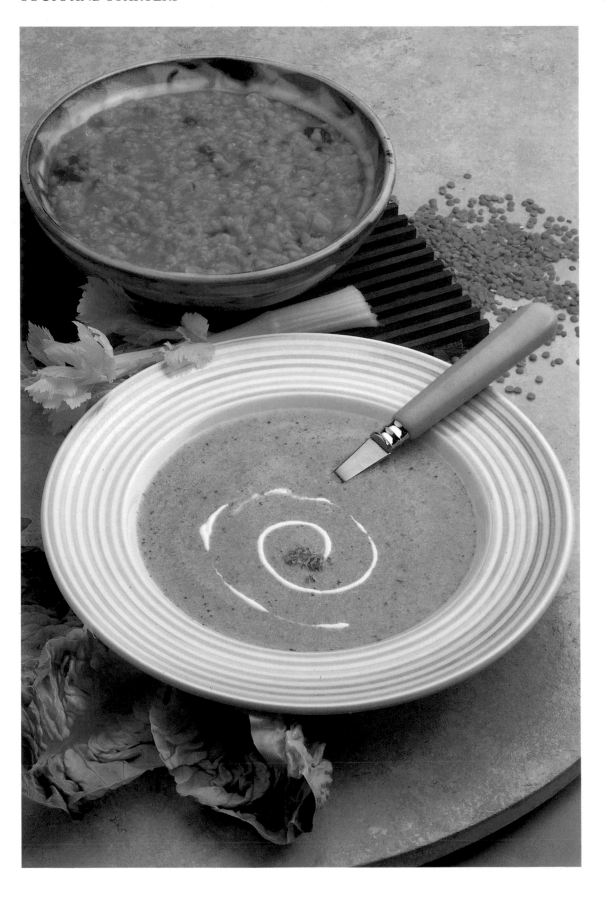

GREEN PEA AND LETTUCE SOUP

50 g/2 oz polyunsaturated margarine
450 g/1 lb shelled fresh or frozen peas
2 lettuce hearts, chopped
1.2 litres/2 pints ham stock or water
1 teaspoon salt
1 teaspoon dried basil
1 teaspoon grated nutmeg
2 bay leaves
TO GARNISH
120 ml/4 fl oz single cream
2 tablespoons chopped parsley

SERVES 8
Per serving:
Energy 110 kcal/450 kJ
CHO 5 g (0.5 units)
Fibre 4 g   **Fat** 8 g   **Protein** 4 g

Melt the margarine in a large saucepan over a low heat. Add the peas (straight from the freezer, if using frozen). Add the chopped lettuce, cover the saucepan and sweat for 10 minutes. Add the stock or water, salt, basil, nutmeg and bay leaves and bring to the boil. Reduce the heat and simmer for 40 minutes. Allow the soup to cool slightly, then remove the bay leaves and transfer the soup to a blender or food processor and purée for about 1 minute. Taste and correct seasoning if necessary.

Reheat the soup and serve piping hot, garnished with a swirl of cream and a sprinkling of parsley.

MELON AND MINT SORBET

600 ml/1 pint water
1 tablespoon lemon juice
2 teaspoons powdered gelatine, soaked in 2 tablespoons cold water
2 sprigs mint, chopped
sugar substitute equivalent to 75 g/3 oz sugar
1 honeydew melon
1 teaspoon peppermint essence
2 egg whites

SERVES 4–6

4 servings
Per serving:
Energy 30 kcal/115 kJ
CHO 5 g (0.5 units)
Fibre 1 g   **Fat** 0 g   **Protein** 1 g

6 servings
Per serving:
Energy 20 kcal/80 kJ
CHO 0 g (0 units)
Fibre 0 g   **Fat** 0 g   **Protein** 1 g

Put the water and lemon juice in a heavy-based pan. Bring to the boil and allow to cool. Add the soaked gelatine and stir until dissolved. Mix in the mint and sweetener. Scoop the flesh from the melon, remove the pips and purée the flesh in a blender. Alternatively, rub through a sieve. Stir into the gelatine mixture with the peppermint essence. Pour mixture into a freezer container and freeze for about 1½ hours or until mushy, stirring occasionally.

Beat the egg whites until they form soft peaks. Fold into the mixture and freeze. Beat the mixture twice at hourly intervals. Cover, seal and freeze.

ABOVE: SPICY LENTIL SOUP (P. 19); BELOW:
GREEN PEA AND LETTUCE SOUP

ICED GRAPEFRUIT

2 large grapefruit
2 oranges, peeled and segmented
1 tablespoon lemon juice
250 ml / 8 fl oz low-calorie lemonade
2 tablespoons finely chopped fresh mint
TO DECORATE
mint sprigs

SERVES 4
Per serving:
Energy 35 kcal / 150 kJ
CHO 10 g (1 unit)
Fibre 1 g **Fat** 0 g **Protein** 0 g

Halve the grapefruit, using a zig-zag cut to give a decorative edge. Remove the flesh from the halves. Remove the membranes from the orange segments and cut the flesh into pieces. Mix with the grapefruit and return to the grapefruit shells.

Mix together the lemon juice, lemonade and mint. Pour into an ice-tray and freeze until mushy. Pile on the grapefruit mixture and decorate each half with a sprig of mint.

TUNA FISH PÂTÉ

2 × 200 g (7 oz) cans tuna fish in brine, drained
    and cut into small pieces
40 g / 1½ oz polyunsaturated margarine
1 tablespoon lemon juice
1 tablespoon grated lemon rind
25 g / 1 oz wholemeal breadcrumbs
salt
freshly ground black pepper

TO GARNISH
lemon wedges
parsley sprig

SERVES 4
Per serving:
Energy 200 kcal / 825 kJ
CHO 5 g (0.5 units)
Fibre 0 g **Fat** 15 g **Protein** 12 g

Place the tuna in a blender with the margarine and blend until smooth. Turn into a bowl and stir in the lemon juice and rind, and breadcrumbs. Mix well, add plenty of salt and pepper. Spoon into a serving dish and garnish with lemon wedges and a sprig of parsley. Serve with toast.

MUSHROOM TERRINE

350 g / 12 oz mushrooms, chopped
175 g / 6 oz minced ham
350 g / 12 oz minced pork
75 g / 3 oz minced onion
40 g / 1½ oz wholemeal breadcrumbs
2 tomatoes, skinned and chopped
1 tablespoon chopped fresh parsley
1 teaspoon chopped fresh thyme

1 large egg
salt and freshly ground pepper

SERVES 8
Per serving:
Energy 120 kcal / 530 kJ
CHO 0 g (0 units)
Fibre 1 g **Fat** 5 g **Protein** 16 g

Place all the ingredients in a bowl and mix together thoroughly. Turn into an earthenware terrine, cover with foil, and bake in a moderately hot oven (190°C, 375°F, Gas Mark 5) for 1–1½ hours. Serve with crusty wholemeal bread.

PRAWN COURGETTES

8 medium courgettes, trimmed
225 g/8 oz peeled prawns
2 tablespoons lemon juice
salt and freshly ground black pepper
25 g/1 oz cottage cheese
1–2 drops liquid sweetener

SERVES 4
Per serving:
Energy 75 kcal/315 kJ
CHO 5 g (0.5 units)
Fibre 1 g **Fat** 1 g **Protein** 12 g

Remove a thin slice lengthways from each courgette. Scoop out the seeds and blanch the courgettes for 3–4 minutes in boiling water. Cool and chill.

Fill with the prawns and sprinkle with 1 tablespoon of lemon juice and pepper. Mix together the cottage cheese, remaining lemon juice and sweetener and season to taste with salt and pepper. When smoothly blended, top each courgette with a little of the cheese mixture. *Illustrated on page 52.*

COURGETTES AND TOMATOES WITH BASIL

750 g/1½ lb courgettes, sliced
salt
1 tablespoon polyunsaturated vegetable oil
1 small onion, chopped
1 garlic clove, crushed
450 g/1 lb tomatoes, skinned and sliced
2 tablespoons wine vinegar
1 tablespoon lemon juice

1 tablespoon chopped fresh basil
freshly ground black pepper

SERVES 4
Per serving:
Energy 80 kcal/335 kJ
CHO 11 g (1 unit)
Fibre 5 g **Fat** 3 g **Protein** 2 g

Sprinkle the courgettes with salt and toss lightly. Leave to drain for 1 hour.

Shake the courgettes in a cloth to dry. Heat the oil in a large frying pan and cook the onion and garlic gently for 5 minutes or until soft. Add the courgettes and cook gently, stirring occasionally, for about 10–15 minutes. When they are soft, add the tomatoes and stir in the vinegar, lemon juice and basil. Add salt and pepper to taste and cook for a further 5 minutes.

Transfer to a warm serving dish.

LEEKS WITH ORANGE AND THYME

3 rashers lean bacon, rinded and chopped
500 g/1¼ lb leeks, trimmed and sliced
4–5 tablespoons orange juice
grated rind of 1 orange
1 tablespoon fresh or 1 teaspoon dried thyme
salt and freshly ground black pepper

SERVES 4
Per serving:
Energy 110 kcal/465 kJ
CHO 10 g (1 unit)
Fibre 2 g **Fat** 6 g **Protein** 4 g

Gently heat the bacon in a frying pan until the fat begins to run. Add the leeks and cook for 2 minutes, stirring constantly.

Make up the orange juice to 150 ml/¼ pint with water, and add to the pan with the rind, thyme, salt and pepper. Bring to the boil and simmer for 10–15 minutes, stirring occasionally until the leeks are just tender and most of the juice has evaporated. *Illustrated on page 93.*

SPICED CAULIFLOWER

2 tablespoons polyunsaturated vegetable oil
2 teaspoons coriander
1 teaspoon ground turmeric
1 cauliflower, divided into florets
2 carrots, scrubbed and thinly sliced
1 large onion, sliced
120 ml/4 fl oz stock
150 ml/¼ pint plain unsweetened yogurt

salt
freshly ground black pepper

SERVES 4
Per serving:
Energy 100 kcal/415 kJ
CHO 8 g (1 unit)
Fibre 2 g   **Fat** 8 g   **Protein** 4 g

Heat the oil in a pan, add the spices and fry gently for 1 minute. Add the vegetables and cook gently for a further 5 minutes.

Add the stock, yogurt, salt and pepper. Stir well, cover and simmer for 10 minutes, or until the vegetables are just tender.

WATERCRESS EGGS

4 eggs, hard-boiled and halved lengthways
salt and freshly ground black pepper
squeeze of lemon juice
2 tablespoons skimmed milk
3–4 tablespoons chopped watercress leaves
lettuce leaves

SERVES 4
Per serving:
Energy 90 kcal/390 kJ
CHO 0 g (0 units)
Fibre 0 g   **Fat** 6 g   **Protein** 7 g

Remove the yolks and mash with salt and pepper. Add the lemon juice, skimmed milk (to give a soft consistency) and water-cress leaves. Press into the white cases and serve on a bed of lettuce.

CRAB AND APPLE COCKTAIL

2 medium crabs or 225 g/8 oz white crab meat
225 g/8 oz crisp apples, peeled, cored and diced
SAUCE
2 tablespoons wine vinegar
150 ml/¼ pint plain unsweetened yogurt
2 tablespoons orange juice
1 tablespoon grated orange rind
½ teaspoon French mustard
2 teaspoons Worcestershire sauce
salt
freshly ground black pepper

TO GARNISH
watercress sprigs
225 g/8 oz crisp apples, unpeeled and thinly sliced
crab legs (optional)

SERVES 4
Per serving:
Energy 130 kcal/560 kJ
CHO 18 g (2 units)
Fibre 2 g   **Fat** 1 g   **Protein** 13 g

Pick the white meat from the crabs and flake it up.

To make the sauce, combine the vinegar, yogurt, orange juice and rind, mustard and Worcestershire sauce. Season to taste.

Mix together the sauce, crab meat and diced apple. Arrange the mixture in scallop shells or individual ramekin dishes or glasses. Garnish with watercress sprigs, slices of apple and crab legs, if available.

CRAB AND APPLE COCKTAIL

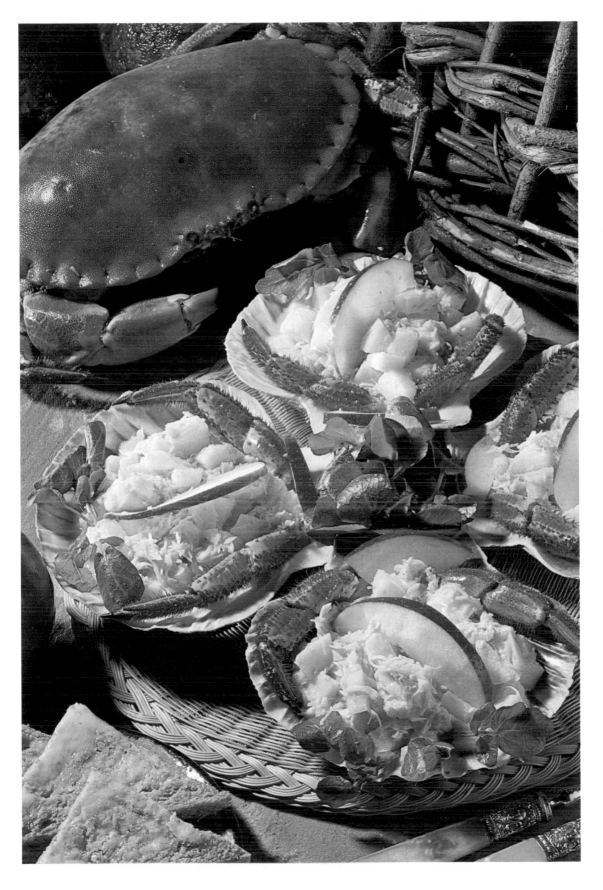

BLACK-EYE FISH

100 g/4 oz black-eye peas, soaked overnight in
  600 ml/1 pint water
225 g/8 oz white fish fillets, cooked, skinned
  and flaked
1 × 100 g (4 oz) can tuna fish, drained and
  flaked
100 g/4 oz peeled prawns
1 small onion, grated
1 tablespoon finely grated lemon rind

2 tablespoons lemon juice
dash of Tabasco sauce
2 teaspoons tomato purée
2 tablespoons chopped parsley
salt
freshly ground black pepper
TO GARNISH
few unshelled prawns
parsley sprigs

**SERVES 4 as a Main Course
        6 as a Starter**

4 servings				6 servings			
Per serving:				**Per serving:**			
Energy 165 kcal/700 kJ				**Energy** 110 kcal/465 kJ			
CHO 0 g (0 units)				**CHO** 0 g (0 units)			
Fibre 1 g	**Fat** 7 g		**Protein** 21 g	**Fibre** 0 g	**Fat** 4 g		**Protein** 14 g

Place the peas and soaking liquid in a pan and bring to the boil. Lower the heat, cover and simmer for 1–1½ hours until the peas are tender, adding more water if necessary.

Drain the peas and place in a bowl. Add the white fish, tuna and prawns and fold lightly to mix. Blend together the remaining ingredients, then fold into the fish mixture. Leave to marinate for at least 1 hour.

Turn into a serving dish, garnish with the prawns and parsley, and serve cold.

CUCUMBER AND COTTAGE CHEESE RING

1 cucumber
300 ml/½ pint hot water
½ teaspoon salt
2 tablespoons powdered gelatine
3 tablespoons lemon juice
450 g/1 lb cottage cheese
250 ml/8 fl oz plain unsweetened yogurt

TO GARNISH
lettuce leaves

SERVES 6

Per serving:		
Energy 30 kcal/135 kJ		
CHO 5 g (0.5 units)		
Fibre 0 g	**Fat** 0 g	**Protein** 3 g

Thinly slice half the cucumber. Place in a saucepan with 150 ml/¼ pint of the water and the salt, and boil gently to soften. Strain, keeping 150 ml/¼ pint of the liquid. Dissolve 1 tablespoon of the gelatine in this liquid and add 1 tablespoon of the lemon juice. Allow to cool.

Arrange the softened cucumber slices in layers in a ring mould and carefully pour over the gelatine mixture. Refrigerate the mould until set.

Dissolve the remaining gelatine in the remaining hot water and add the remaining lemon juice and a little salt. Leave to cool. Peel and chop the remaining cucumber. Blend the cottage cheese and yogurt together and stir in the cooled gelatine mixture and the chopped cucumber. Pour over the cucumber in the ring mould and chill until firm.

Serve turned out on a bed of lettuce leaves on a serving platter.

Salads

NAPOLEON'S BEAN SALAD

225 g/8 oz dried haricot beans, soaked
  overnight in cold water
1 onion, quartered
1 carrot, scraped and quartered
1 bouquet garni
salt and freshly ground black pepper
4 tablespoons finely chopped fresh herbs
2 tablespoons lemon juice

1 tablespoon tarragon vinegar
1 teaspoon prepared French mustard

SERVES 6
Per serving:
Energy 110 kcal/460 kJ
CHO 20 g (2 units)
Fibre 10 g   **Fat** 0 g   **Protein** 8 g

Drain the beans and put them in a large pan or casserole. Add the onion, carrot, bouquet garni and plenty of black pepper. Pour over sufficient water to cover the beans by 1 cm/½ inch. Cook in a preheated cool oven (150°C, 300°F, Gas Mark 2) for 3 hours, or simmer on top of the stove for 2–3 hours. Replace the water if necessary, so that the beans do not dry out.

Season the cooked beans to taste with salt and cook for a further 5 minutes. Drain, then remove and discard the onion, carrot and bouquet garni. Place the beans in a large serving bowl. Add the chopped herbs, lemon juice, vinegar and mustard. Stir to mix and chill for about 1 hour.

MIXED BEAN SALAD

225 g/8 oz French beans, halved
450 g/1 lb broad beans, shelled
1 × 425 g (15 oz) can butter beans, drained
1 × 425 g (15 oz) can cannellini beans, drained
DRESSING
4 tablespoons polyunsaturated vegetable oil
2 tablespoons wine vinegar
1 tablespoon chopped fresh mint
salt
freshly ground black pepper
TO GARNISH
1 hard-boiled egg, finely chopped

SERVES 4–5
4 servings
Per serving:
Energy 370 kcal/1560 kJ
CHO 45 g (4.5 units)
Fibre 19 g   **Fat** 13 g   **Protein** 21 g

6 servings
Per serving:
Energy 295 kcal/1250 kJ
CHO 35 g (3.5 units)
Fibre 15 g   **Fat** 10 g   **Protein** 17 g

Cook the French beans and broad beans together in boiling, salted water for 5 minutes. Drain, then mix with the rinsed butter beans and cannellini beans.

Put all the dressing ingredients in a screw-topped jar and shake well. Pour the dressing over the beans while they are still warm, then leave the salad to cool. Chill for 30 minutes. Scatter the chopped egg over the surface of the salad before serving.

TUNA BEAN SALAD

*225 g/8 oz frozen broad beans, cooked and
    cooled*
*1 × 425 g (15 oz) can red kidney beans, drained
    and rinsed under cold running water*
*1 × 200 g (7 oz) can tuna fish, drained and
    roughly flaked*
2 tablespoons chopped fresh chives
1 × 5 cm/2 inch piece cucumber, diced
4 celery sticks, sliced
*1 dessert apple, unpeeled, quartered, cored and
    chopped*
1 tablespoon grated lemon rind
2 tablespoons lemon juice
lettuce leaves (optional)
TO GARNISH
lemon slices
cucumber slices

SERVES 4
Per serving:
Energy 290 kcal/1215 kJ
CHO   25 g (2.5 units)
Fibre 12 g **Fat** 11 g **Protein** 22 g

Put the broad beans and kidney beans in a
bowl with the tuna fish, chives, cucumber
and celery. Toss the apple and lemon rind
in the lemon juice and mix thoroughly
with the other ingredients. Serve in a salad
bowl. If preferred the salad may be arranged on a bed of crisp lettuce. Garnish
with lemon and cucumber slices.

VARIATION
Use 175 g/6 oz dried, red kidney beans
instead of canned. Soak the beans overnight, drain and cook them in unsalted
boiling water for 2–2½ hours, boiling
rapidly for the first 10 minutes to get rid of
toxins, until well cooked.

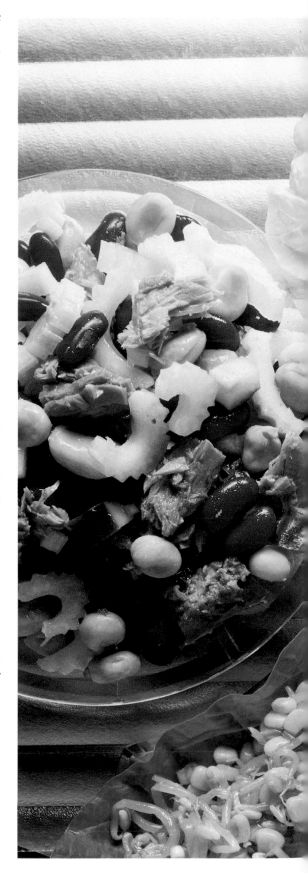

CLOCKWISE FROM THE TOP: RED BEAN AND
CARROT SALAD (P. 30); COTTAGE CHEESE
SALAD (P. 30); SWEETCORN AND BEAN-
SPROUT SALAD (P. 30); TUNA BEAN SALAD

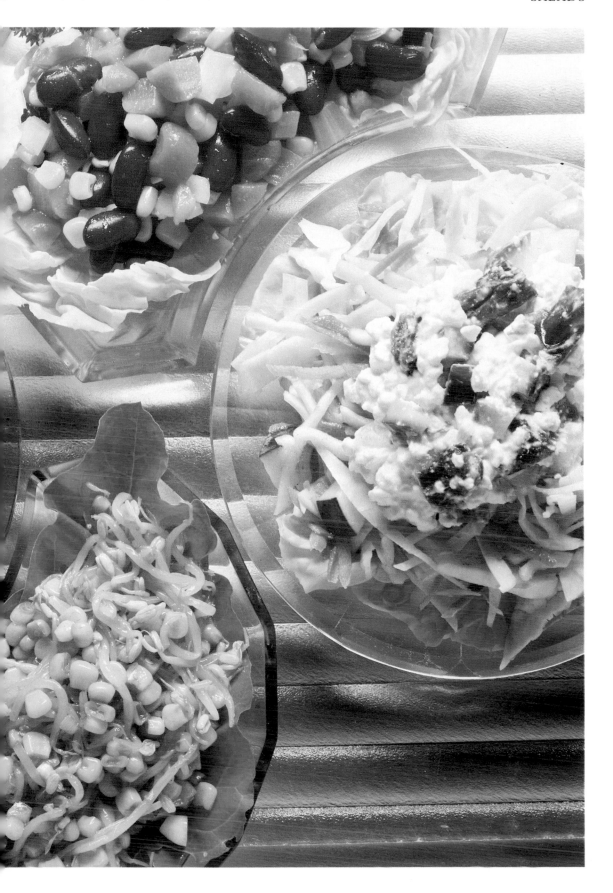

RED BEAN AND CARROT SALAD

1 × 200 g (7 oz) can sweetcorn kernels, drained
1 × 425 g (15 oz) can red kidney beans, drained
    and rinsed under cold running water
1 tablespoon finely chopped onion
225–350 g/8–12 oz carrots, scraped, diced and
    cooked
4 tablespoons French dressing
salt

freshly ground black pepper
lettuce leaves

SERVES 6
Per serving:
Energy 170 kcal/710 kJ
CHO   18 g (2 units)
Fibre   9 g   **Fat** 7 g   **Protein** 6 g

Mix together all the ingredients, except the lettuce, seasoning to taste with salt and pepper. Spoon on to a bed of lettuce to serve. *Illustrated on page 29.*

COTTAGE CHEESE SALAD

450 g/1 lb cottage cheese
1 × 7.5 cm (3 inch) piece cucumber, diced
225 g/8 oz dates, stoned
350 g/12 oz white cabbage, or Chinese leaves,
    cored and shredded
2 large carrots, scraped and coarsely grated
4 spring onions, chopped, or 1 tablespoon grated
    onion
2 red dessert apples, unpeeled, cored and chopped
2 tablespoons lemon juice

lettuce leaves
TO GARNISH
parsley sprigs

SERVES 6
Per serving:
Energy 165 kcal/685 kJ
CHO   22 g (2 units)
Fibre   3 g   **Fat** 3 g   **Protein** 11 g

Put the cottage cheese and cucumber into a bowl. Reserve four dates for the garnish; roughly chop the remainder and mix with the cheese. Combine the cabbage or Chinese leaves and onions. Dip the apples in the lemon juice, then fold into the mixture.

Arrange a bed of lettuce leaves on a flat serving dish and top with the cabbage mixture, keeping it flat. Spoon the cottage cheese mixture across the centre and garnish with the reserved dates and parsley. *Illustrated on page 29.*

SWEETCORN AND BEAN-SPROUT SALAD

1 × 300 g (11 oz) can sweetcorn kernels, drained
1 × 300 g (11 oz) can bean-sprouts, drained, or
    225 g/8 oz fresh bean-sprouts, blanched for 1
    minute and drained
8 spring onions, chopped
1 tablespoon soy sauce
salt and freshly ground black pepper
spinach leaves, torn into pieces

SERVES 6
Per serving:
Energy 50 kcal/215 kJ
CHO   9 g (1 unit)
Fibre   5 g   **Fat** 0 g   **Protein** 2 g

Mix together all the ingredients, except the spinach. Season to taste with salt and pepper. Line a salad bowl with the spinach and spoon the sweetcorn salad on top. *Illustrated on page 29.*

BROAD BEAN AND HAM SALAD

175 g/6 oz thick-cut ham, cubed
1 tablespoon Worcestershire sauce
500 g/1¼ lb shelled broad beans
150 ml/¼ pint plain unsweetened yogurt
1 teaspoon chopped fresh chives
large pinch of paprika
½ teaspoon salt
freshly ground black pepper
lettuce leaves

TO GARNISH
chopped chives

SERVES 4
Per serving:
Energy 130 kcal/560 kJ
CHO 10 g (1 unit)
Fibre 5 g   **Fat** 3 g   **Protein** 15 g

Mix the ham with the Worcestershire sauce. Leave for 10 minutes. Cook the beans in boiling water for 5 minutes. Drain and refresh under cold running water. Add to the ham with the yogurt, chives, paprika, salt and pepper. Mix well.

Line a shallow salad dish with the lettuce leaves and spoon over the beans and ham mixture. Chill for 30 minutes before serving, garnished with chives.

SUMMER SALAD

450 g/1 lb small new potatoes, washed and unpeeled
2 dessert apples, unpeeled, cored and diced
2 celery sticks, chopped
1 pear, unpeeled, cored and diced
225 g/8 oz cherries, stoned and halved
100 g/4 oz cottage cheese
150 ml/¼ pint plain unsweetened yogurt

TO GARNISH
mint sprigs

SERVES 4
Per serving:
Energy 190 kcal/805 kJ
CHO 38 g (4 units)
Fibre 5 g   **Fat** 1 g   **Protein** 8 g

This dish combines well with a green salad and wholemeal rolls.

Cook the potatoes in boiling water. Drain, allow to cool and cut into dice.

Place the diced potatoes in a bowl and combine with the remaining ingredients. Mix well. Turn into a serving bowl and garnish with sprigs of mint.

LENTIL SALAD

175 g/6 oz green lentils, soaked for 1 hour in cold water
1 tablespoon lemon juice
1 tablespoon vinegar
1 garlic clove, crushed
salt
4 spring onions, chopped
4 tomatoes, chopped

2 celery sticks, chopped
freshly ground black pepper

SERVES 4
Per serving:
Energy 145 kcal/620 kJ
CHO 25 g (2.5 units)
Fibre 6 g   **Fat** 0 g   **Protein** 11 g

Cook the lentils in slightly salted water for 30–40 minutes or until tender. Drain well and mix with the lemon juice and vinegar, garlic and salt, while still warm. Add the remaining ingredients and mix thoroughly.

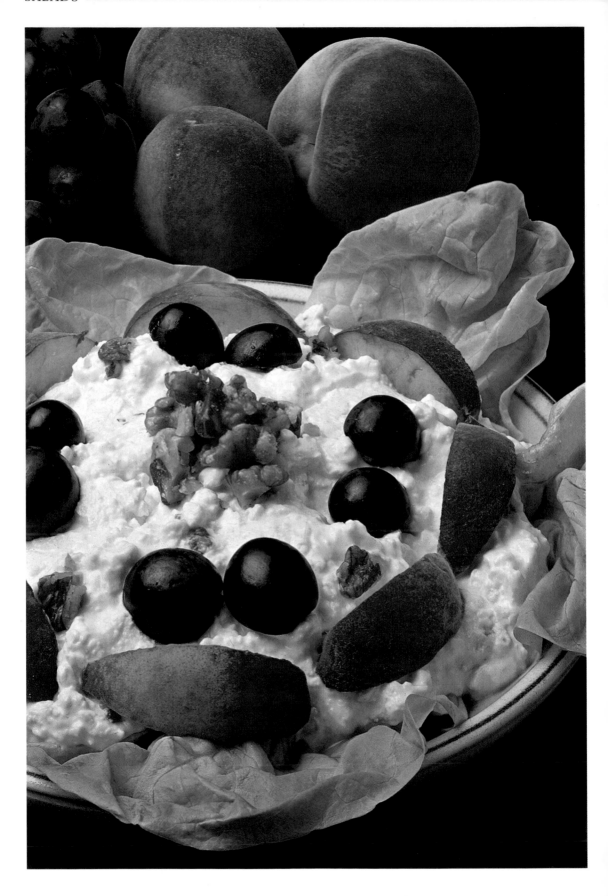

COURGETTE AND CHIVE SALAD

350 g / 12 oz courgettes
1 tablespoon polyunsaturated vegetable oil
2 tablespoons lemon juice
salt and freshly ground black pepper
1 tablespoon chopped fresh chives

SERVES 4
Per serving:
Energy 50 kcal / 200 kJ
CHO 0 g (0 units)
Fibre 1 g **Fat** 3 g **Protein** 0 g

Place the courgettes in a large pan of lightly salted boiling water and cook for 5 minutes. Drain and rinse in cold water. Cut the courgettes crossways into 1 cm / ½ inch slices and place in a shallow serving dish.

Mix together the oil, lemon juice, salt and pepper and pour over the courgettes. Sprinkle with the chopped chives and chill for about 30 minutes before serving.

WALDORF SALAD

450 g / 1 lb red dessert apples, unpeeled and cored
2 tablespoons lemon juice
150 ml / ¼ pint plain unsweetened yogurt
½ head celery, chopped
50 g / 2 oz walnuts, chopped
1 lettuce, separated into leaves

SERVES 4
Per serving:
Energy 140 kcal / 590 kJ
CHO 16 g (2 units)
Fibre 3 g **Fat** 6 g **Protein** 3 g

Slice one apple thinly and dice the remainder. Dip the apple slices in a dressing made with the lemon juice and 1 tablespoon of the yogurt. Set aside. Toss the diced apple in the remaining dressing and let it stand for 30 minutes.

Add the celery and walnuts to the diced apples with the rest of the yogurt and mix thoroughly. Line a serving bowl with the lettuce leaves, pile the salad in the centre and garnish with the apple slices.

CHEESE AND FRUIT SALAD

225 g / 8 oz cottage cheese
3 tablespoons plain unsweetened yogurt
lettuce leaves
1 fresh peach, or canned unsweetened sliced peaches
TO GARNISH
8 black grapes or black olives
chopped walnuts

SERVES 2
Per serving:
Energy 155 kcal / 645 kJ
CHO 11 g (1 unit)
Fibre 1 g **Fat** 0 g **Protein** 17 g

Blend together the cottage cheese and yogurt. Arrange lettuce leaves around the edge of a serving dish and pile the cottage cheese mixture in the centre. Arrange the sliced peaches over the cottage cheese. Garnish with black grapes or black olives and chopped walnuts.

CHEESE AND FRUIT SALAD

TOSSED GREEN SALAD

½ lettuce, separated into leaves
½ bunch curly endive
½ bunch watercress, washed
¼ cucumber, sliced
1 green pepper, cored, seeded and sliced
few spring onions
2 tablespoons French dressing

SERVES 4
Per serving:
Energy 55 kcal/235 kJ
CHO 0 g (0 units)
Fibre 0 g **Fat** 5 g **Protein** 0 g

Put all the vegetables into a deep salad bowl. Pour over the dressing and toss well.

ORANGE AND MINT SALAD

4 large oranges, peel and pith removed
2 tablespoons finely chopped mint
4 tablespoons lemon juice
6 tablespoons wine vinegar
artificial sweetener
salt
freshly ground black pepper

TO GARNISH
mint sprigs

SERVES 4
Per serving:
Energy 40 kcal/160 kJ
CHO 8 g (1 unit)
Fibre 2 g **Fat** 0 g **Protein** 1 g

Cut the orange flesh into thin slices. Place in a serving dish and sprinkle with the mint. Mix the lemon juice with the vinegar, adding sweetener to taste. Season with salt and pepper and pour over the orange and mint. Garnish with mint.

MELON AND CHICKEN SALAD

4 tablespoons plain unsweetened yogurt
pinch of garlic powder (optional)
salt
freshly ground black pepper
1 tablespoon chopped chives
2 tablespoons chopped mint
350 g/12 oz cooked chicken, cut into narrow
    strips
1 honeydew melon, seeded and cut into cubes or
    thin slices

lettuce leaves
TO GARNISH
2 tomatoes, cut into wedges
sprig of fresh mint

SERVES 4
Per serving:
Energy 160 kcal/685 kJ
CHO 8 g (1 unit)
Fibre 2 g **Fat** 4 g **Protein** 25 g

Mix together the yogurt and garlic powder (if using). Season to taste with salt and pepper, then stir in the chives and mint. Add the chicken and melon and mix lightly. Cover and leave the salad to stand for about 20 minutes before serving.

Arrange the lettuce on a serving platter and pile the salad on top. Garnish with tomato wedges and a sprig of fresh mint.

MELON AND CHICKEN SALAD

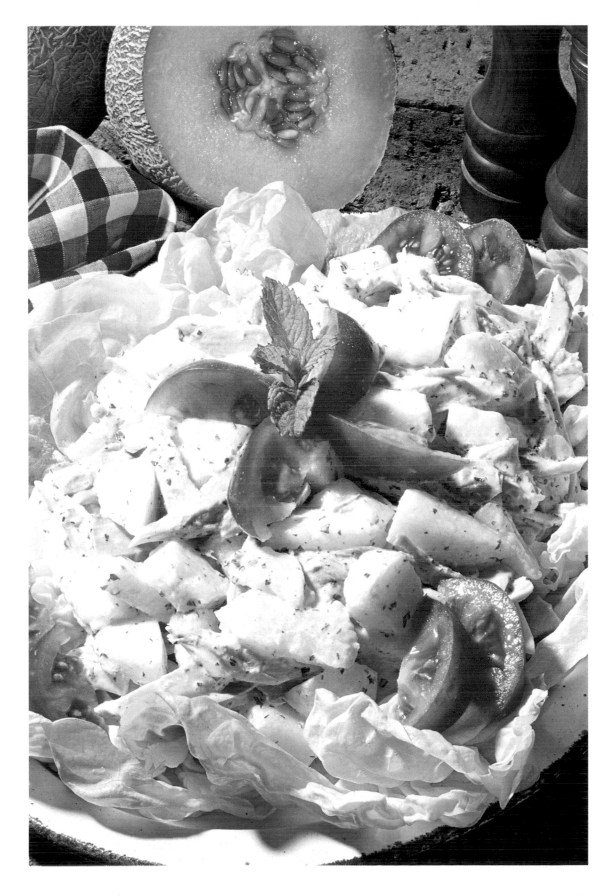

LENTIL SALAD WITH WALNUTS

225 g/8 oz red lentils, rinsed thoroughly
3 spring onions, finely chopped
2 tablespoons finely chopped fresh parsley
1 garlic clove, crushed
salt
freshly ground black pepper
1 tablespoon white wine vinegar
3 tablespoons plain unsweetened yogurt

2 bacon rashers, rinded, grilled until crisp and
  chopped
2 tablespoons finely chopped walnuts

SERVES 4
Per serving:
Energy 280 kcal/1180 kJ
CHO 30 g (3 units)
Fibre 7 g **Fat** 9 g **Protein** 19 g

Discard any discoloured lentils. Cook the lentils in boiling water for about 30 minutes or until tender but not mushy. Drain the lentils thoroughly.

Mix together the spring onions, parsley, garlic, salt and pepper to taste, vinegar and yogurt. Mix in the cooked lentils, bacon and half the walnuts. Spoon into a serving dish and sprinkle with the remaining walnuts. This salad is delicious served while it is still warm.

APPLE AND CABBAGE SLAW

1 medium head of white cabbage, finely
  shredded
4 red apples, unpeeled, cored and thinly sliced
1 tablespoon lemon juice
1 small green pepper, cored, seeded and diced
1 medium onion, finely sliced
120 ml/4 fl oz plain unsweetened yogurt
25 g/1 oz Edam cheese, grated

SERVES 6
Per serving:
Energy 65 kcal/280 kJ
CHO 11 g (1 unit)
Fibre 2 g **Fat** 1 g **Protein** 3 g

Place the cabbage in a large bowl. Sprinkle the apple slices with lemon juice to prevent them from going brown. Add to the cabbage with the diced pepper, onion and yogurt. Toss lightly. Sprinkle with the grated cheese.

ORANGE AND CHICORY SALAD

4 heads chicory, cut crossways into 5 mm/¼
  inch thick slices
3 oranges, peeled, pith removed and thinly
  sliced across the segments
4 tablespoons polyunsaturated vegetable oil
2 tablespoons orange juice
salt
freshly ground black pepper

SERVES 4
Per serving:
Energy 170 kcal/700 kJ
CHO 7 g (1 unit)
Fibre 1 g **Fat** 14 g **Protein** 1 g

Put the chicory and orange slices in a serving bowl. Shake together the oil, orange juice, salt and pepper in a screw-topped jar. Pour this dressing over the chicory and orange slices. Toss the ingredients lightly and serve at once.

RED CABBAGE SALAD

2 dessert apples, unpeeled, cored and sliced
450 g / 1 lb red cabbage, finely shredded
1 bunch watercress, washed and sprigged
2 tablespoons sultanas
DRESSING
3 tablespoons polyunsaturated vegetable oil
1 tablespoon vinegar
1 garlic clove, crushed
½ teaspoon French mustard
salt

freshly ground black pepper
TO GARNISH
chopped parsley

SERVES 4
Per serving:
Energy 160 kcal / 665 kJ
CHO 13 g (1 unit)
Fibre 5 g **Fat** 11 g **Protein** 2 g

To prepare the dressing, mix the oil, vinegar, garlic, mustard, salt and pepper in a screw-topped jar and shake well.

Pour this dressing over the apples in a bowl and toss to coat them completely.

Mix in the cabbage, watercress and sultanas. Toss well and serve sprinkled with the chopped parsley.

WINTER SALAD

4 medium potatoes, cooked and diced
1 large celery stick, finely chopped
2 carrots, scraped and grated
1 small onion, finely chopped
½ small white cabbage, shredded
8 black olives, stoned and chopped
120 ml / 4 fl oz plain unsweetened yogurt

TO GARNISH
2 tablespoons finely chopped parsley

SERVES 4
Per serving:
Energy 85 kcal / 355 kJ
CHO 15 g (1.5 units)
Fibre 2 g **Fat** 1 g **Protein** 2 g

Put the potatoes, celery, carrots, onion, cabbage and olives in a salad bowl. Pour over the yogurt and toss well.

Sprinkle the salad with the chopped parsley and serve.

MIXED SPRING SALAD WITH HERB DRESSING

3 tablespoons finely chopped fresh mixed herbs
4 tablespoons French dressing
1 garlic clove, crushed
salt
freshly ground black pepper
1 lettuce, shredded
1 bunch watercress, cleaned and trimmed
4 spring onions, washed and diced

TO GARNISH
spring onions, cleaned and trimmed

SERVES 6
Per serving:
Energy 70 kcal / 290 kJ
CHO 0 g (0 units)
Fibre 0 g **Fat** 6 g **Protein** 0 g

Mix together the herbs, dressing, garlic and salt and pepper to taste. Leave to stand for 2 hours. In a large bowl mix together the lettuce, watercress and spring onions. Pour over the dressing and serve garnished with the whole spring onions.

STRAWBERRY SALAD

1 small cucumber, peeled and thinly sliced
12 large strawberries, hulled and thinly sliced
pinch of salt
freshly ground black pepper
2 tablespoons dry white wine

SERVES 4
Per serving:
Energy 20 kcal/75 kJ
CHO 4 g (0.5 units)
Fibre 1 g **Fat** 0 g **Protein** 0 g

Arrange the cucumber and strawberry slices decoratively on a shallow serving dish: an outer circle of cucumber, slightly overlapped by a circle of strawberry slices, then more cucumber, with strawberry slices in the centre. Sprinkle over the salt, pepper and wine and chill for about 20 minutes before serving.

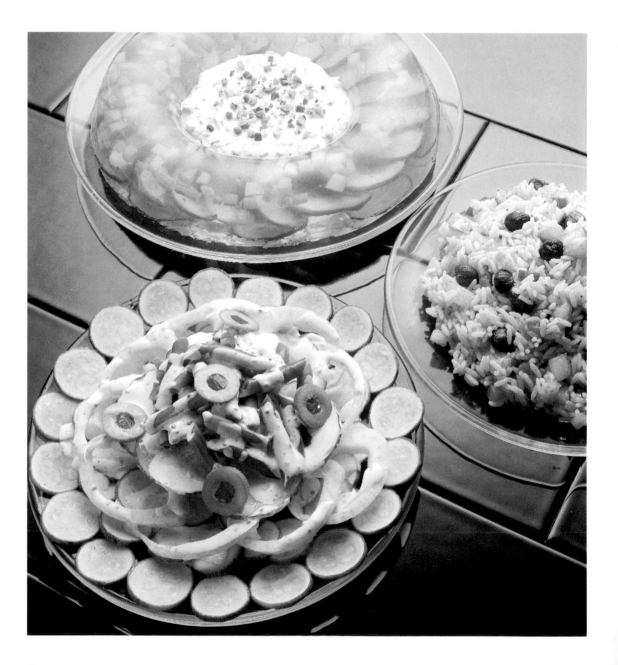

FENNEL SALAD

175–225 g/6–8 oz courgettes, thinly sliced
salt
1 large fennel, thinly sliced
¼ cucumber, thinly sliced
225 g/8 oz French beans, sliced and cooked

150 ml/¼ pint plain unsweetened yogurt
1 tablespoon mustard with seeds
TO GARNISH
6 stuffed green olives, sliced

SERVES 4–6
4 servings
Per serving:
Energy 50 kcal/200 kJ
CHO 5 g (0.5 units)
Fibre 2 g **Fat** 1 g **Protein** 3 g

6 servings
Per serving:
Energy 30 kcal/140 kJ
CHO 0 g (0 units)
Fibre 1 g **Fat** 0 g **Protein** 2 g

Put the courgette slices on a plate, sprinkle with salt and leave for 15 minutes to draw out the excess moisture.

Wash and thoroughly dry the courgette slices and place them in the bottom of a salad bowl. Arrange the fennel on top, then the cucumber and finally the beans.

Mix the yogurt with the mustard and pour it over the salad. Garnish with the sliced olives, and chill the salad for 30 minutes before serving.

FRUIT AND NUT RICE SALAD

225 g/8 oz brown rice
12 whole cardamom seeds
salt
1 × 200 g (7 oz) can unsweetened pineapple rings, drained and roughly chopped
½ cucumber, diced
50 g/2 oz hazelnuts, roasted
DRESSING
2 tablespoons grated orange rind

4 tablespoons orange juice
4 tablespoons polyunsaturated vegetable oil
2 teaspoons curry paste

SERVES 6
Per serving:
Energy 260 kcal/1100 kJ
CHO 38 g (4 units)
Fibre 1 g **Fat** 11 g **Protein** 3 g

Cook the rice with the cardamom seeds in boiling, salted water for 10–15 minutes or until the rice is just tender. Drain the rice and run cold water through the grains to remove any excess starch. Mix the chopped pineapple into the rice with the cucumber and hazelnuts.

Put all the dressing ingredients into a screw-topped jar and shake together well. Stir the dressing through the rice salad so that it is evenly coated.

CLOCKWISE FROM THE TOP: AMERICAN MOULD (P. 76); FENNEL SALAD; FRUIT AND NUT RICE SALAD

Main Course Dishes

TURKEY NUT LOAF

1 medium onion, finely chopped
100 g/4 oz walnuts, chopped
750 g/1½ lb raw turkey meat, minced
175 g/6 oz wholemeal breadcrumbs
1 tablespoon Worcestershire sauce
½ teaspoon chopped fresh mixed herbs or ¼
   teaspoon dried mixed herbs
1 tablespoon chopped parsley
1 egg
salt
freshly ground black pepper

TO GARNISH
1 × 425 g (15 oz) can unsweetened apricot
   halves, drained
stuffed olives, sliced
lettuce leaves

SERVES 8
Per serving:
Energy 440 kcal/1820 kJ
CHO 15 g (1.5 units)
Fibre 5 g   **Fat** 28 g   **Protein** 30 g

Blend all the ingredients together with plenty of salt and pepper. Spoon the mixture into a well greased 1 kg (2 lb) loaf tin and cover with greased foil. Bake in a preheated moderate oven (180°C, 350°F, Gas Mark 4) for 1½ hours. Cool in the pan for 30 minutes, then turn out and allow to become quite cold.

Arrange some of the apricot halves over the top of the loaf. Any leftover can be added to a salad to serve with the loaf. Place the olives on the top edges of the loaf. Garnish with lettuce.

OVEN-COOKED PILAFF

350 g/12 oz boneless raw chicken, finely diced
600 ml/1 pint chicken stock
25 g/1 oz polyunsaturated margarine
25 g/1 oz flaked almonds
1 tablespoon pine nuts (optional)
225 g/8 oz brown rice
½ teaspoon ground ginger
¼ teaspoon ground cinnamon

salt and freshly ground black pepper
2 bay leaves

SERVES 4
Per serving:
Energy 400 kcal/1720 kJ
CHO 15 g (1.5 units)
Fibre 2 g   **Fat** 11 g   **Protein** 22 g

Place the diced chicken in a saucepan and pour over the chicken stock. Bring to the boil, reduce the heat, cover and simmer for 5 minutes.

Heat the margarine in a clean saucepan and use to fry the flaked almonds and pine nuts, then the rice, stirring until the rice is transparent. Sprinkle in the ground ginger and cinnamon and stir for 1 minute. Add the strained stock from cooking the chicken and bring to the boil. Remove from the heat, stir in the diced chicken. Season with salt and pepper and pour the mixture into a greased shallow casserole. Lay the bay leaves on top. Cover and cook in a moderately hot oven (190°C, 375°F, Gas Mark 5) for 35 minutes, or until all the liquid has been absorbed.

CHICKEN BAKE WITH YOGURT TOPPING

15 g/½ oz polyunsaturated margarine
1 small onion, finely chopped
2 celery sticks, finely chopped
100 g/4 oz button mushrooms
350 g/12 oz cooked chicken, finely chopped
1 tablespoon chopped parsley
freshly ground black pepper
TOPPING
300 ml/½ pint plain unsweetened yogurt

2 egg yolks
1 teaspoon prepared mustard

SERVES 4
Per serving:
Energy 270 kcal/1120 kJ
CHO 5 g (0.5 units)
Fibre 1 g **Fat** 13 g **Protein** 31 g

Melt the margarine in a frying pan. Add the onion, celery and mushrooms and cook gently for 5 minutes, stirring frequently. Add the chicken, parsley and pepper to taste, then transfer the mixture to a casserole and press down firmly.

To make the topping: put the yogurt in a bowl with the egg yolks, mustard and salt and pepper to taste. Mix well, then pour over the chicken. Bake in a preheated moderately hot oven (190°C, 375°F, Gas Mark 5) for 25 minutes. Serve hot. *Illustrated on page 42.*

CHICKEN AND VEGETABLE FRICASSÉE

4 chicken portions (about 150 g/5 oz each, with bone)
3 onions, finely chopped
1 garlic clove, crushed
2 celery sticks, thinly sliced
2 carrots, scraped and thinly sliced
1 bay leaf
150 ml/¼ pint chicken stock
1 teaspoon chopped thyme
1 teaspoon paprika

freshly ground black pepper
TO GARNISH
chopped parsley

SERVES 4
Per serving:
Energy 130 kcal/540 kJ
CHO 0 g (0 units)
Fibre 1 g **Fat** 3 g **Protein** 22 g

Take a piece of fat from the chicken and rub over the base of a heavy pan. Put in the chicken and cook gently over a very low heat until golden on all sides. Add the onions and garlic and continue cooking gently for 3 minutes, stirring occasionally.

Add the remaining ingredients, cover and cook over a low heat for 1¼ hours or until the chicken is tender. Taste and adjust the seasoning. Sprinkle with parsley and serve hot. *Illustrated on page 42.*

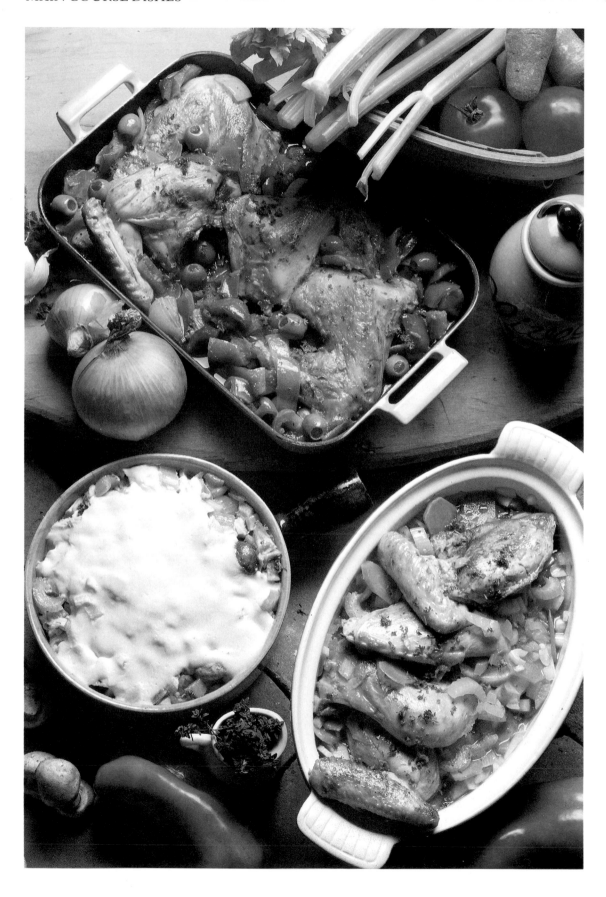

CHICKEN AND OLIVE BAKE

4 chicken portions (about 150 g/5 oz each, with
  bone)
5 tablespoons cider vinegar
4 tomatoes, chopped
2 green peppers, cored, seeded and chopped
2 onions, chopped
1 small garlic clove, crushed
1 teaspoon chopped marjoram
freshly ground black pepper
a little polyunsaturated vegetable oil

2 tablespoons tomato purée
75 g/3 oz stuffed olives
TO GARNISH
chopped thyme

SERVES 4
Per serving:
Energy 150 kcal/630 kJ
CHO 5 g (0.5 units)
Fibre 2 g **Fat** 8 g **Protein** 16 g

Arrange the chicken portions in a shallow dish. Mix together the vinegar, tomatoes, peppers, onions, garlic, marjoram and pepper to taste. Pour over the chicken. Leave to marinate for 2 hours, turning the chicken once.

Heat the oil in a deep frying pan. Drain the chicken, reserving the marinade. Add the chicken to the pan and fry until browned on all sides. Stir in the reserved marinade with the tomato purée and the olives. Cover and simmer over a low heat for 1 hour. Taste and adjust seasoning, sprinkle with thyme and serve hot.

BOILED CHICKEN AND PASTA

25 g/1 oz polyunsaturated margarine
2 onions, chopped
2 garlic cloves, crushed
3 celery sticks, chopped
1.75 kg/4 lb boiling chicken with giblets
salt and freshly ground black pepper
1 bay leaf
1 tablespoon dried oregano
175–225 g/6–8 oz wholemeal pasta (any kind)

2 tablespoons grated Parmesan cheese
TO GARNISH
tomato wedges

SERVES 4
Per serving:
Energy 520 kcal/2190 kJ
CHO 40 g (4 units)
Fibre 2 g **Fat** 16 g **Protein** 57 g

Melt the margarine in a saucepan. Add the onions, garlic and celery and cook until softened. Add the chicken with its giblets, cover with water and bring to the boil. Skim. Season with salt and pepper to taste and add the bay leaf. Simmer gently for 2–2½ hours or until cooked.

Remove the chicken from the pan and allow to cool slightly, then remove the skin. Take the meat from the bones and dice it. Strain the cooking stock into another saucepan and add the oregano and pasta. Cook until tender. Strain the stock back into the first saucepan, and reheat the chicken in this. Drain the hot chicken and pile on to a warmed serving dish. Surround with the pasta and sprinkle over the Parmesan. Garnish with tomato wedges.

CLOCKWISE FROM THE TOP: CHICKEN AND OLIVE BAKE: CHICKEN AND VEGETABLE FRICASSÉE (P. 41); CHICKEN BAKE WITH YOGURT TOPPING (P. 41)

CURRIED CHICKEN WITH CORIANDER

1 onion, halved
1 carrot, scraped and coarsely chopped
1 celery stick, coarsely chopped
1.5 kg/3½ lb roasting chicken
1 bay leaf
3 sprigs parsley
3 sprigs lovage
1 teaspoon sea salt
6 black peppercorns
SAUCE
3 tablespoons desiccated coconut
25 g/1 oz polyunsaturated margarine
1 large onion, finely chopped
2 garlic cloves, crushed
1 tablespoon mild curry powder
¼ teaspoon ground turmeric

¼ teaspoon ground cumin seed
¼ teaspoon ground coriander
pinch of ground chilli
3 tablespoons lemon juice
1 tablespoon wholemeal flour
4 tablespoons plain unsweetened yogurt
2 tablespoons chopped almonds
2 tablespoons chopped coriander or 3 tablespoons
   chopped basil

SERVES 4
Per serving:
Energy 500 kcal/2100 kJ
CHO 10 g (1 unit)
Fibre 4 g   **Fat** 24 g   **Protein** 60 g

Put the vegetables in a saucepan with the chicken, bay leaf, parsley, lovage, salt and peppercorns. Pour in enough cold water just to cover the chicken and poach for 1 hour, or 20 minutes in a pressure cooker. Lift out the chicken when it is tender. When the chicken is cool enough to handle, remove all the skin and bones and cut the meat into neat small pieces. Set aside.

Strain the liquid in which the chicken was cooked, discarding the vegetables and herbs. Taste the stock: if it is too weak, reduce it by fast boiling until it has a good flavour. Measure off 600 ml/1 pint.

To make the sauce, pour 300 ml/½ pint of the stock over the desiccated coconut in a bowl and leave for 15 minutes to form a coconut 'milk'. Melt the margarine in a large saucepan and cook the onion gently until pale golden, adding the garlic halfway through. Sprinkle on the curry powder and spices, stirring all the time. Pour on the remaining stock and stir until blended. Simmer gently for 15 minutes, then add the lemon juice. Pour the coconut 'milk' through a sieve into the curry sauce, pushing lightly with the back of a wooden spoon to extract all the liquid. Stir the flour into the yogurt to make a smooth paste and add it to the curry sauce, continuing to stir until all is blended. Add the chicken pieces to the sauce. Reheat, stirring and finally add the almonds and the coriander (or basil). Stand, covered, for 5 minutes before serving. Accompany with plain boiled rice.

CHICKEN AND ORANGE CASSEROLE

2 medium onions, quartered
2 celery sticks, sliced
4 chicken portions (about 150 g/5 oz each, with
   bone), skinned
1 tablespoon chopped fresh herbs
3 tablespoons grated orange rind
5 tablespoons orange juice
150 ml/¼ pint chicken stock
salt and freshly ground black pepper

TO GARNISH
1 orange, thinly sliced
watercress

SERVES 4
Per serving:
Energy 210 kcal/890 kJ
CHO 7 g (1 unit)
Fibre 1 g   **Fat** 6 g   **Protein** 32 g

Blanch the onions and celery in boiling water for 2 minutes. Put the chicken, celery and onion into a casserole, sprinkle over the herbs, orange rind and juice, and the stock. Add salt and pepper to taste.

Cover tightly and cook in a preheated moderate oven (180°C, 350°F, Gas Mark 4) for about 1 hour, until the chicken is tender. Serve garnished with orange slices and watercress.

BARBECUE BEANS AND CHICKEN

4 chicken legs, washed and dried
salt
2 teaspoons paprika
1 tablespoon wholemeal flour
2 tablespoons polyunsaturated vegetable oil
1 × 425 g (15 oz) can red kidney beans, drained
40 g / 1½ oz polyunsaturated margarine
1 onion, chopped
1 tablespoon vinegar
½ teaspoon chilli powder

3 tablespoons tomato purée
85 ml / 3 fl oz plain unsweetened yogurt
TO GARNISH
parsley sprigs

SERVES 4
Per serving:
Energy 380 kcal/1600 kJ
CHO 20 g (2 units)
Fibre 9 g   **Fat** 18 g   **Protein** 33 g

Season the chicken legs with salt and 1 teaspoon of the paprika and coat with the flour. Heat the oil in a frying pan and fry the chicken quickly until golden brown. Transfer to a medium casserole. Add the kidney beans.

Melt the margarine in a small pan, add the onion and cook for 5 minutes. Add the vinegar, chilli powder and remaining paprika. Mix the tomato purée with the yogurt and add to the pan, stirring well to combine. Bring to the boil, then pour the sauce over the chicken and beans. Cook in a preheated moderately hot oven (200°C, 400°F, Gas Mark 6) for about 20 minutes. Serve garnished with parsley.

CHICKEN PAPRIKA

4 chicken portions (about 150 g / 5 oz each, with bone)
1 teaspoon salt
2 teaspoons paprika
150 ml / ¼ pint chicken stock
1 onion, finely chopped
150 ml / ¼ pint plain unsweetened yogurt
freshly ground black pepper

TO GARNISH
2 tablespoons finely chopped parsley

SERVES 4
Per serving:
Energy 130 kcal/550 kJ
CHO 0 g (0 unit)
Fibre 0 g   **Fat** 4 g   **Protein** 20 g

Sprinkle the chicken portions with the salt and paprika pepper. Put in a grill pan, without the rack, and cook under a preheated grill for 5 minutes on each side, or until well browned. (Do not put too near the heat or they will scorch before browning.) Remove and place in a lidded casserole with the chicken stock and the onion. Cover and simmer over a moderate heat for 30–40 minutes or until tender.

adding more stock if necessary. Lift out the chicken portions, place on a warmed serving dish and keep hot. If there is excess liquid, reduce to 150 ml / ¼ pint. Stir in the yogurt and adjust the seasoning. Heat slowly, stirring well, but do not allow to boil. Pour over the chicken and sprinkle with chopped parsley.

CHICKEN AND HAM MOULD

1 tablespoon powdered gelatine
3 tablespoons water
2 × 425 g (15 oz) cans chicken soup
1 teaspoon Worcestershire sauce
salt and freshly ground black pepper
1 × 185 g (6½ oz) can pimientoes, drained and
   chopped
50 g/2 oz lean ham, cubed
100 g/4 oz cooked chicken, chopped
1 × 10 cm (4 inch) piece of cucumber, cut into
   5 mm/¼ inch cubes

TO GARNISH
pimiento strips
cucumber slices

SERVES 4
Per serving:
Energy 140 kcal/590 kJ
CHO 8 g (1 unit)
Fibre 1 g   **Fat** 7 g   **Protein** 12 g

Sprinkle the gelatine over the water in a heatproof bowl, then place over a pan of gently simmering water. Stir until dissolved. Mix together the soup, Worcestershire sauce and gelatine mixture. Season to taste with salt and pepper. Add the pimientoes, ham, chicken and cucumber. Mix well and pour into a 1.2 litre (2 pint) mould. Leave to set, before turning out on to a serving platter. Garnish with strips of pimiento and cucumber slices.

LEMON CHICKEN

5–6 Chinese mushrooms, soaked in tepid water
   for 20 minutes
1 chicken, weighing 1.5–2 kg/3–4½ lb, boned
   and cut into 2.5 cm/1 inch cubes
1 teaspoon salt
freshly ground black pepper
3 tablespoons polyunsaturated vegetable oil
4 slices root ginger, chopped
1 red pepper, cored, seeded and chopped
1 tablespoon grated lemon rind
5 spring onions, thinly sliced

4 tablespoons dry sherry
2 tablespoons soy sauce
1 teaspoon cornflour, blended with 1 tablespoon
   water
1–2 tablespoons lemon juice

SERVES 6
Per serving:
Energy 290 kcal/1230 kJ
CHO 5 g (0.5 units)
Fibre 1 g   **Fat** 14 g   **Protein** 34 g

Squeeze the mushrooms dry and remove the hard stalks, then shred the mushroom caps.

Mix the chicken with salt and pepper to taste and ½ tablespoon of the oil. Heat the remaining oil in a wok or frying pan. Add the chicken and stir-fry for 2 minutes. Remove from the pan and keep warm. Add the ginger, red pepper and mushrooms to the pan and stir-fry for 1 minute. Add the lemon rind and spring onions and fry for 30 seconds. Sprinkle in the sherry and soy sauce and bring to the boil, then stir in the blended cornflour. Return the chicken to the pan and cook, stirring, for 1 minute. Sprinkle with the lemon juice and serve hot.

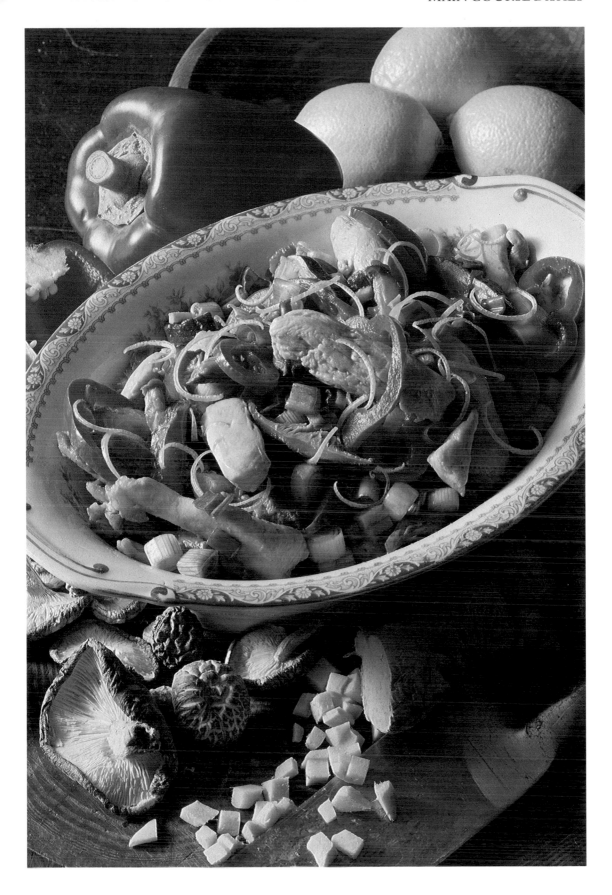

ORANGE-STUFFED TURKEY OLIVES

4 turkey escalopes (about 120 g/4½ oz each)
polyunsaturated vegetable oil for frying
STUFFING
50 g/2 oz fresh, wholemeal breadcrumbs
1 tablespoon grated orange rind
8 stuffed olives, sliced
40 g/1½ oz cooked ham, chopped
salt and freshly ground black pepper
25 g/1 oz polyunsaturated margarine
1 small onion, finely chopped
SAUCE
15 g/½ oz polyunsaturated margarine
1 onion, chopped
1 garlic clove, crushed
2 teaspoons wholemeal flour

3 tablespoons orange juice
150 ml/¼ pint water or stock
1 × 275 g (10 oz) can sweetcorn, mashed
TO GARNISH
stuffed olive slices
orange slices
parsley sprigs

SERVES 4
Per serving:
Energy 295 kcal/1235 kJ
CHO   22 g (2 units)
Fibre   6 g   **Fat** 16 g   **Protein** 17 g

Place the turkey escalopes between two pieces of cling film and beat until thin.

To make the stuffing, mix together the breadcrumbs, orange rind, olives, ham and salt and pepper to taste. Melt the margarine in a pan and cook the onion for 5 minutes. Stir into the stuffing to bind it together.

Divide the stuffing between the escalopes and roll up, securing with cocktail sticks. Heat the oil in a pan and fry the turkey olives gently for 10–15 minutes, turning occasionally, until almost cooked through. Remove with a slotted spoon and place in a shallow ovenproof dish. Cook in a preheated moderate oven (180°C, 350°F, Gas Mark 4) for 15 minutes.

To make the sauce, heat the margarine in a pan, add the onion and garlic and cook gently for 5 minutes. Stir in the flour and cook for 1 minute. Gradually blend in the orange juice and water or stock. Stir in the corn and add salt and pepper to taste. Heat through gently and pour over the turkey olives. Return to the oven for 15 minutes. Serve hot, garnished with olives, orange slices and parsley.

MONKS' MACKEREL

4 medium mackerel, cleaned and gutted
2 onions, chopped
2 bay leaves
4 tablespoons lemon juice
2 teaspoons dried mixed herbs
12 black olives, stoned
salt
freshly ground black pepper

TO GARNISH
watercress sprigs
lemon wedges

SERVES 4
Per serving:
Energy 280 kcal/1160 kJ
CHO   0 g (0 units)
Fibre   2 g   **Fat** 21 g   **Protein** 19 g

Place the mackerel in a non-stick baking dish and cover with the onions, bay leaves, lemon juice, herbs and stoned olives. Season with salt and pepper. Cover with foil and bake in a preheated moderate oven (180°C, 350°F, Gas Mark 4) for 30–40 minutes or until the fish is cooked. Serve hot garnished with the watercress sprigs and lemon wedges.

MONKS' MACKEREL

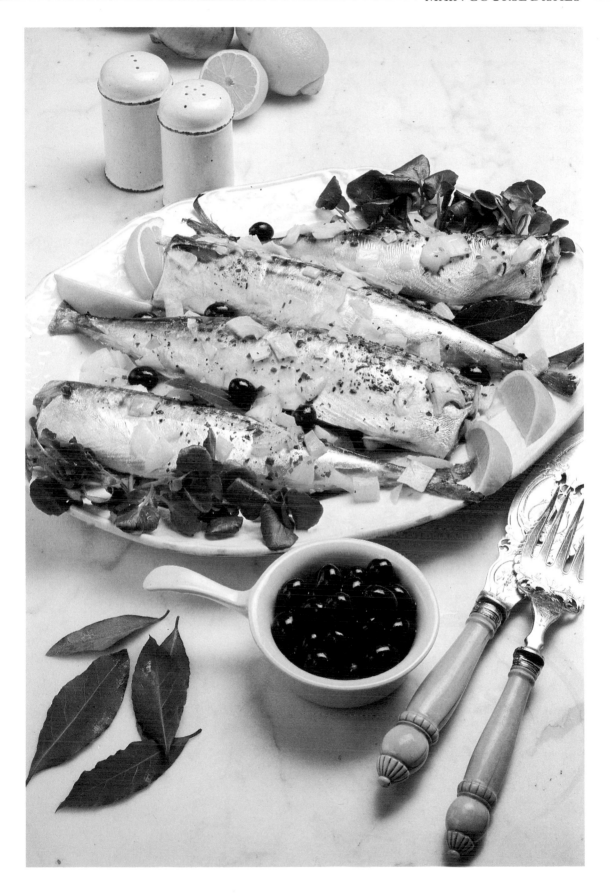

COD AND BEAN PIE

175 g/6 oz haricot beans, soaked overnight in
   cold water
2 medium onions, chopped
1 kg/2 lb cod or other white fish fillets, skinned
   and cut into small pieces
4 rashers streaky bacon, rinded and cut into
   strips
salt
freshly ground black pepper
pinch of dried thyme
pinch of dried marjoram

600 ml/1 pint milk or milk and fish stock,
   mixed
450 g/1 lb potatoes, very thinly sliced
TO GARNISH
1 tablespoon chopped parsley

SERVES 6
Per serving:
Energy 345 kcal/1460 kJ
CHO   30 g (3 units)
Fibre   8 g   **Fat** 8 g   **Protein** 37 g

Drain the haricot beans, cover with fresh cold water, bring to the boil and simmer for 1½ hours or until tender. Drain.

Put the onions into a greased casserole and cover with the fish and strips of bacon. Season to taste and add the herbs. Add a layer of cooked beans and pour in the milk or milk and stock. Top with the potatoes which should overlap and be arranged to form an attractive crust. Bake in a pre-heated moderate oven (180°C, 350°F, Gas Mark 4) for about 40 minutes or until the potatoes are cooked and golden brown. Sprinkle the parsley over the pie and serve it very hot.

COD AND PINEAPPLE KEBABS

1 × 425 g (15 oz) can unsweetened pineapple
   chunks
120 ml/4 fl oz light soy sauce
4 tablespoons dry sherry
1 tablespoon grated fresh root ginger
1 teaspoon dry mustard
1 garlic clove, crushed
900 g/2 lb cod, cut into 2.5 cm/1 inch cubes

1 green pepper, cored, seeded and cut into
   2.5 cm/1 inch squares

SERVES 6
Per serving:
Energy 155 kcal/645 kJ
CHO   13 g (1 unit)
Fibre   1 g   **Fat** 2 g   **Protein** 22 g

Drain the pineapple, reserving 4 table-spoons of the liquid. Mix the reserved liquid with the soy sauce, sherry, ginger, mustard and garlic in a shallow dish. Add the fish cubes and turn to coat. Cover and leave to marinate for at least an hour.

Drain the fish cubes, reserving the marinade. Thread the fish cubes, pineapple and green pepper on to skewers. Cook under a preheated grill (or over charcoal) 10–13 cm (4–5 inch) from the source of heat, for 8–10 minutes, or until the fish flakes easily, when tested with a fork. Turn and baste with the marinade during cooking. Serve hot with rice.

PRAWN AND PINEAPPLE KEBABS

120 ml / 4 fl oz soy sauce
120 ml / 4 fl oz dry sherry
2 teaspoons sesame oil
1 tablespoon minced fresh root ginger
1 garlic clove, crushed
450 g / 1 lb large prawns, peeled (about 24)
½ fresh pineapple, peeled, cored and cut into
   wedges
450 g / 1 lb Brussels sprouts

salt
2 red peppers, cored, seeded and cut into 2.5 cm /
   1 inch squares

SERVES 4
Per serving:
Energy 250 kcal / 1040 kJ
CHO   9 g (1 unit)
Fibre   5 g   **Fat** 8 g   **Protein** 27 g

Combine the soy sauce, sherry, sesame oil, root ginger and garlic in a shallow bowl. Place the prawns and pineapple chunks in the mixture and leave to marinate for 3–4 hours, turning occasionally.

Blanch the Brussels sprouts in boiling salted water for 1–2 minutes, drain.

Drain the prawns and pineapple, reserving the marinade. Thread the prawns, pineapple, Brussels sprouts and peppers on to four metal skewers, alternating ingredients, ending with a sprout. Brush with the reserved marinade and grill under a preheated grill for 3–4 minutes, turning once and brushing with the marinade. Grill until the fish is just cooked through.

SEAFOOD CURRY

25 g / 1 oz polyunsaturated margarine
1 small onion, chopped
1 teaspoon curry powder
2 teaspoons wholemeal flour
150 ml / ¼ pint plain unsweetened yogurt
1 small dessert apple, unpeeled, cored and
   chopped
225 g / 8 oz peeled prawns
2 tomatoes, skinned, seeded and chopped

salt and freshly ground black pepper
TO GARNISH
lemon wedges

SERVES 4
Per serving:
Energy 140 kcal / 570 kJ
CHO   10 g (1 unit)
Fibre   1 g   **Fat** 5 g   **Protein** 12 g

Melt the margarine in a saucepan, add the onion and cook gently for 3 minutes or until soft and golden, stirring occasionally. Stir in the curry powder and flour and cook for 2 minutes.

Remove from the heat and stir in the yogurt, apple and prawns. Return to the heat and cook gently for 5 minutes. Add the tomatoes and continue cooking for 3 minutes. Add salt and pepper to taste. Garnish with lemon wedges. Serve hot with brown rice.

POACHED WHITING IN PIQUANT SAUCE

4 whiting fillets, washed and wiped
275 ml / 9 fl oz plain unsweetened yogurt
2 teaspoons prepared mustard
4 teaspoons lemon juice
salt
freshly ground black pepper
4 tablespoons finely chopped parsley
TO GARNISH
lemon slices

SERVES 4
Per serving:
Energy 135 kcal / 570 kJ
CHO 5 g (0.5 units)
Fibre 0 g **Fat** 1 g **Protein** 24 g

Poach the fish in a little water or stock until tender. Meanwhile mix together the yogurt, mustard and lemon juice in a small bowl. Heat over a saucepan of hot water, but do not allow to boil. Taste and adjust the seasoning with salt and pepper and stir in the parsley. Spoon over the cooked fish and garnish with the lemon slices.

CLOCKWISE FROM THE TOP: BAKED STUFFED HADDOCK; POACHED WHITING IN PIQUANT SAUCE; PRAWN COURGETTES (P. 23)

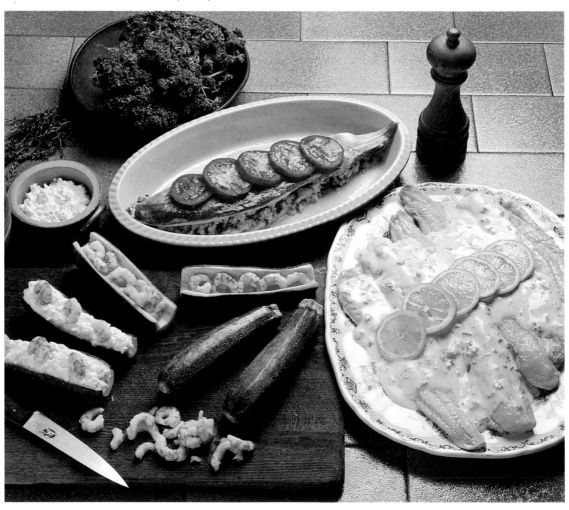

BAKED STUFFED HADDOCK

2 haddock fillets, about 350 g/12 oz each,
   washed and dried
2 slices wholemeal bread, crumbed
3 tablespoons finely chopped parsley
1/4 teaspoon finely grated lemon rind
1/2 teaspoon thyme
1/2 teaspoon salt
white pepper
25 g/1 oz polyunsaturated margarine, melted

milk
2 large tomatoes, sliced

SERVES 4
Per serving:
Energy 195 kcal/810 kJ
CHO 5 g (0.5 units)
Fibre 1 g **Fat** 7 g **Protein** 26 g

Place one haddock fillet, skin side down, in a greased shallow heatproof dish. Make a stuffing by combining the breadcrumbs with 1 tablespoon of the parsley, the lemon rind, thyme, salt and pepper, and binding loosely with 15 g/1/2 oz of the margarine and a little milk. Cover the fish with the stuffing. Put the second fillet, skin side uppermost, on top of the stuffing. Arrange a line of tomato slices along the centre. Sprinkle with the remaining parsley. Coat with the remaining margarine and bake, uncovered, in a preheated moderate oven (180°C, 350°F, Gas Mark 4) for 40 minutes.

FISH LASAGNE

350 g/12 oz cod fillets, skinned
600 ml/1 pint semi-skimmed milk
salt
freshly ground black pepper
8 sheets wholemeal lasagne (about 175 g/6 oz)
50 g/2 oz polyunsaturated margarine
1 onion, chopped
100 g/4 oz mushrooms, chopped
1 red pepper, cored, seeded and chopped

1 × 200 g (7 oz) can tuna fish, drained
50 g/2 oz wholemeal flour
50 g/2 oz Cheddar cheese, grated

SERVES 4
Per serving:
Energy 540 kcal/2260 kJ
CHO 20 g (2 units)
Fibre 4 g **Fat** 30 g **Protein** 40 g

Place the cod in a saucepan, pour on only enough milk to cover and add salt and pepper. Bring to the boil, cover and simmer gently for 8–10 minutes or until tender. Leave to cool.

Bring a large pan of salted water to the boil. Cook the lasagne, four sheets at a time, for about 11 minutes or until just tender. Drain and place on a cloth to dry.

Melt 25 g/1 oz of the margarine in a pan and fry the onion until soft. Add the mushrooms and pepper and continue cooking for 2–3 minutes, then set aside.

Drain the cod and make the liquid up to 600 ml/1 pint with the remaining milk, and set on one side. Flake the cod, removing any remaining bones, and mix with the flaked tuna fish.

Melt the remaining margarine in a pan, stir in the flour and cook for 1 minute. Gradually add the milk, stirring continuously, bring to the boil and cook for 2 minutes. Add salt and pepper. Stir three-quarters of the sauce into the mushroom mixture.

Place two sheets of lasagne in a greased shallow casserole to cover the bottom. Cover with one-third of the fish and one-third of the mushroom mixture. In this way continue layering the rest of the lasagne, fish and mushroom mixture, finishing with a layer of lasagne. Pour the remaining white sauce over the lasagne and sprinkle with grated cheese. Cook in a preheated moderately hot oven (200°C, 400°F, Gas Mark 6) for about 40 minutes.

VEAL AND ORANGE CASSEROLE

1 tablespoon polyunsaturated vegetable oil
1 medium onion, finely chopped
2 tablespoons finely grated orange rind
3–4 fresh sage leaves, finely chopped
275 g/10 oz lean boneless veal, cut into 2.5 cm/
*   1 inch cubes*
wholemeal flour
salt and freshly ground black pepper
150 ml/¼ pint chicken stock
150 ml/¼ pint dry vermouth
3 tablespoons orange juice

TO GARNISH
chopped sage (optional)
grated orange rind (optional)

SERVES 2
Per serving:
Energy 390 kcal/1650 kJ
CHO 10 g (1 unit)
Fibre 0 g   **Fat** 18 g   **Protein** 29 g

Heat the oil in a heavy saucepan or flame-proof casserole. Add the onion and fry gently for 3 minutes. Add the orange rind and sage leaves and cook gently for 1 minute.

Dust the cubed veal in flour, season with salt and pepper, and add to the onion mixture. Fry steadily until the veal is sealed on all sides. Gradually stir in the stock, vermouth and orange juice. Cover and simmer gently for about 1 hour or until the veal is tender. Taste and adjust the seasoning before serving. Garnish with more chopped fresh sage or grated orange rind.

GINGERED BEEF WITH TURNIP

1.25 kg/2½ lb stewing beef, in two pieces
3 slices root ginger
1 teaspoon black peppercorns
120 ml/4 fl oz soy sauce
2 tablespoons dry sherry
1 kg/2 lb turnips, peeled and cut into 1 cm/½
*   inch thick slices*
2 teaspoons cornflour, blended with 2
*   tablespoons water*

TO GARNISH
chopped parsley

SERVES 8
Per serving:
Energy 315 kcal/1325 kJ
CHO 10 g (1 unit)
Fibre 4 g   **Fat** 17 g   **Protein** 33 g

Put the beef into a saucepan with the ginger, peppercorns, soy sauce and sherry. Add enough water just to cover the meat and bring to the boil. Cover and simmer for 1 hour or until tender. Meanwhile, parboil the turnips for 2 minutes, then drain well.

Remove the beef from the pan and cut into 1 cm/½ inch thick slices. Put the slices of beef into a deep, heatproof bowl and arrange the turnips on top. Pour the liquid from the pan over the turnips and steam for 30 minutes. Drain the liquid from the bowl into a saucepan, discarding the ginger. Arrange the beef and turnips in a warmed serving dish and keep hot.

Add the blended cornflour to the pan and simmer, stirring, until thickened. Pour over the beef and turnips and serve garnished with parsley.

FARMHOUSE BEEF AND SWEETCORN STEW

15 g/½ oz polyunsaturated margarine
450 g/1 lb stewing beef, cubed
2 large onions, chopped
1 carrot, peeled and chopped
600 ml/1 pint stock
salt
freshly ground black pepper
1 teaspoon ground paprika
1 × 350 g (12 oz) can sweetcorn

1 × 65 g (2½ oz) can tomato purée
150 ml/¼ pint plain unsweetened yogurt

SERVES 4
Per serving:
Energy 265 kcal/1115 kJ
CHO 20 g (2 units)
Fibre 5 g   Fat 8 g   Protein 28 g

Melt the margarine in a flameproof casserole, add the beef and brown on all sides. Add the onions and carrot and cook for about 5 minutes. Gradually add the stock, blending well. Season with salt and pepper to taste and the paprika. Cover and cook in a preheated moderate oven (160°C, 325°F, Gas Mark 3) for 1–1¼ hours or until the beef is tender.

Add the sweetcorn with the can juice, mixing well. Cover and cook for a further 30 minutes, stirring occasionally. Add the tomato purée, blending well. Reheat gently on top of the cooker but do not allow to boil. Add the yogurt and serve immediately.

LAMB AND BARLEY STEW

1 tablespoon polyunsaturated vegetable oil
750 g/1½–1¾ lb boned shoulder of lamb, cut into 5 cm/2 inch cubes
25 g/1 oz pearl barley, soaked for 2 hours in cold water
50 g/2 oz unsoaked dried apricots
few parsley stalks
25 g/1 oz sultanas
1 onion, sliced
1 garlic clove, crushed
450 ml/1¾ pint stock

1 tablespoon lemon juice
salt
freshly ground black pepper
TO GARNISH
chopped parsley

SERVES 4
Per serving:
Energy 470 kcal/1930 kJ
CHO 15 g (1.5 units)
Fibre 4 g   Fat 26 g   Protein 44 g

Heat the oil in a frying pan, add the lamb in batches and fry until browned on all sides. Transfer to a flameproof casserole with a slotted spoon. Drain the pearl barley and add to the casserole, with the apricots, parsley stalks and sultanas.

Add the onion and garlic to the fat remaining in the frying pan and fry gently for 5 minutes without browning. Stir in the stock, lemon juice and salt and pepper to taste and bring to the boil, then pour over the lamb.

Place the casserole over a moderate heat and bring to the boil. Lower the heat, cover and simmer for 1 hour or until the lamb is tender, stirring occasionally.

LAMB KEBABS WITH BARBECUE SAUCE

*450 g / 1 lb lean lamb, cut into 4 cm / 1½ inch
    cubes*
8 small tomatoes, washed
12 small mushrooms, cleaned and trimmed
5 tablespoons lemon juice
3 tablespoons soy sauce
4 teaspoons Worcestershire sauce
1 garlic clove, crushed
40 g / 1½ oz polyunsaturated margarine
TO FINISH
½ small cabbage, washed and shredded
4 carrots, grated
2 small apples, washed, unpeeled and diced

SERVES 4
Per serving:
Energy   310 kcal / 1310 kJ
CHO   10 g (1 unit)
Fibre   5 g   **Fat** 18 g   **Protein** 27 g

Thread the meat, tomatoes and mush-rooms alternately on to four skewers. Put the lemon juice, soy sauce, Worcestershire sauce, garlic and margarine into a small pan and heat to melt the fat. Marinate the skewered kebabs in the mixture for at least 2 hours.

Cook the kebabs on a barbecue or under a preheated hot grill for 10–15 minutes or until the meat is tender, turning and basting with the remaining sauce. Serve on a bed of shredded cabbage, carrot and apple with the remainder of the barbecue sauce.

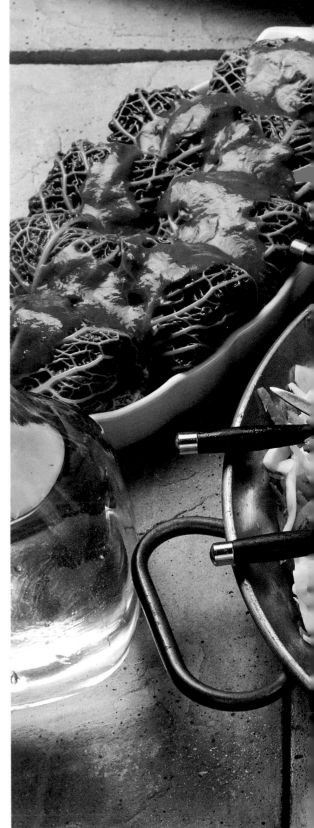

LEFT: DOLMAS (P. 90); RIGHT: LAMB KEBABS WITH BARBECUE SAUCE

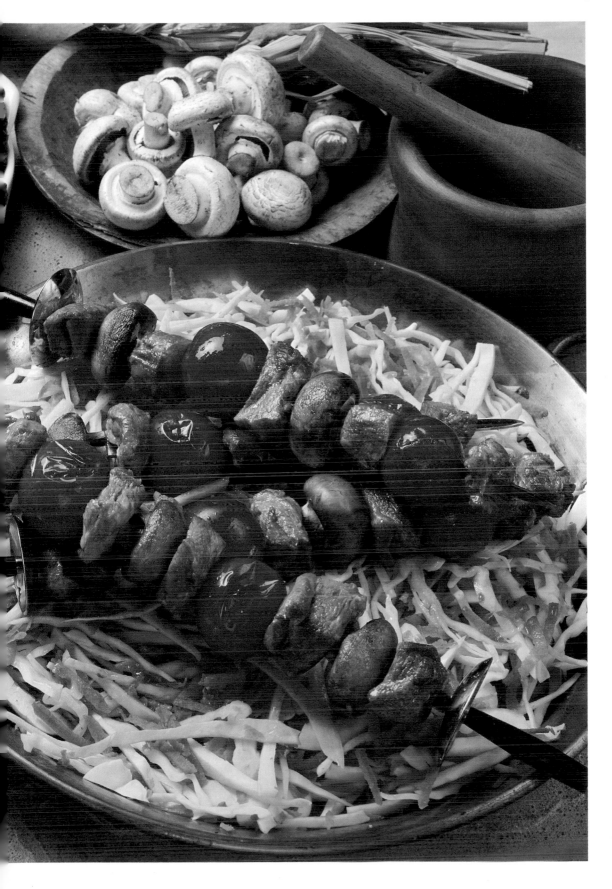

PORK CHOPS IN ORANGE SAUCE

4 pork chops (about 150 g/5 oz each), trimmed
salt
freshly ground black pepper
2 teaspoons dried sage
25 g/1 oz polyunsaturated margarine
1 garlic clove, crushed
15 g/½ oz cornflour
300 ml/½ pint chicken stock
6 tablespoons orange juice

2 fresh oranges, peeled, pith removed and
   segmented
TO GARNISH
watercress

SERVES 4
Per serving:
Energy 400 kcal/1730 kJ
CHO 10 g (1 unit)
Fibre 1 g   **Fat** 29 g   **Protein** 29 g

Season the chops with salt and pepper and sprinkle sage over each one. Heat the margarine in a pan and fry the garlic for 1 minute, then brown the chops on both sides. Remove and leave on one side. Stir the cornflour into the remaining fat in the pan and cook for a few minutes. Gradually add the stock and orange juice and bring to the boil. Return the chops to the pan, reduce the heat, add the segments from 1 of the oranges, cover and cook for about 40 minutes. Taste the sauce and adjust the seasoning.

Place the chops on a serving plate with orange segments. Pour sauce over and serve garnished with segments from the remaining orange and watercress.

STUFFED PEPPERS

4 even-size peppers
175 g/6 oz streaky bacon, rinded and chopped
1 onion, chopped
100 g/4 oz wholemeal breadcrumbs
1 medium cooking apple, peeled, cored and
   chopped
25 g/1 oz walnuts, chopped
1 teaspoon mixed dried herbs
salt
freshly ground black pepper

1 egg, beaten
1 tablespoon polyunsaturated vegetable oil
2–3 tablespoons water

SERVES 4
Per serving:
Energy 335 kcal/1400 kJ
CHO 15 g (1.5 units)
Fibre 4 g   **Fat** 25 g   **Protein** 11 g

Cut off the stalk end of each pepper and reserve. Carefully remove the core and all the seeds without breaking the sides. Stand the peppers in a deep dish. Cover with boiling water and leave for 5 minutes while preparing the filling.

Fry the bacon over a medium heat and as soon as the fat starts to run, add the onion and cook until softened. Remove the pan from the heat and stir in the breadcrumbs, apple, walnuts, herbs, salt and pepper. Mix in enough of the beaten egg to make a firm, moist mixture.

Drain the peppers well and stand them in a deep, well-greased dish. Spoon in the filling, replace the reserved stalk ends and brush with the oil. Add the water to the dish, cover with foil or a lid and cook in a preheated moderately hot oven (190°C, 375°F, Gas Mark 5) for about 35 minutes or until the peppers are tender.

PORK AND CABBAGE CASSEROLE

1 bouquet garni
120 g/4½ oz peeled chestnuts
750 g/1½–1¾ lb boned pork shoulder, weighed
    after fat trimmed
1 large potato, peeled and quartered
2 medium onions, quartered
4 medium carrots, scraped
1 tablespoon tomato purée
2 tablespoons white wine vinegar
600 ml/1 pint light stock

salt
freshly ground black pepper
2 bay leaves
225 g/8 oz red cabbage, thinly sliced

SERVES 4
Per serving:
Energy 380 kcal/1600 kJ
CHO 20 g (2 units)
Fibre 6 g   **Fat** 15 g   **Protein** 41 g

Put all the ingredients, except the red cabbage, into a large flameproof casserole. Bring to the boil, lower the heat, cover and simmer for about 1½ hours or until the pork has become tender.

Add the cabbage, increase the heat and cook for a further 5 minutes.

STUFFED MARROW

15 g/½ oz polyunsaturated margarine
1 small onion, chopped
2 rashers streaky bacon, rinded
15 g/½ oz wholemeal flour
1 × 400 g (14 oz) can tomatoes
150 ml/¼ pint cold water
1 teaspoon horseradish sauce
pinch of nutmeg
bay leaf
salt
freshly ground black pepper
1 medium marrow, cut in half lengthways, seeds
    removed
STUFFING
1 tablespoon polyunsaturated vegetable oil

1 large onion, chopped
225 g/8 oz cooked pork, minced
100 g/4 oz wholemeal breadcrumbs
1 garlic clove, crushed (optional)
1 teaspoon dried basil
1 tablespoon grated lemon rind
1 tablespoon lemon juice
salt
freshly ground black pepper

SERVES 6
Per serving:
Energy 200 kcal/860 kJ
CHO 10 g (1 unit)
Fibre 4 g   **Fat** 11 g   **Protein** 15 g

To make the sauce, melt the margarine, add the onion and bacon and fry gently for 1 minute. Stir in the flour, then, off the heat, blend in the tomatoes and their juice with the water. Stirring all the time, bring the sauce to the boil, then mix in the horseradish sauce, nutmeg, bay leaf, salt and pepper. Simmer, uncovered, for 15 minutes. Rub the sauce through a sieve or liquidize in a blender. Taste and adjust the seasoning.

Place the marrow in a pan of boiling salted water and cook gently for 5 minutes. Drain well and arrange in a lightly greased ovenproof dish.

To make the stuffing, heat the oil in a pan. Add the onion and fry gently until golden brown. Stir in the pork, breadcrumbs, garlic, basil, lemon rind and juice and plenty of salt and pepper. Bind the ingredients together with 4 tablespoons of the tomato sauce, then divide the filling between the marrow halves, packing it well down. Bake in a preheated moderately hot oven (200°C, 400°F, Gas Mark 6) uncovered, for 20–25 minutes. Heat the remaining tomato sauce and serve it in a separate bowl.

BUTTER BEAN, HERB AND TOMATO SOUFFLÉ

100 g / 4 oz butter beans, soaked overnight in
   600 ml / 1 pint water
150 ml / ¼ pint milk
1 large onion, grated
4 tomatoes, skinned and chopped
1 tablespoon chopped parsley
1 tablespoon dried thyme
1 teaspoon chopped sage
salt
freshly ground black pepper
3 eggs, separated

SERVES 4–6
4 servings
Per serving:
Energy 170 kcal/720 kJ
CHO 20 g (2 units)
Fibre 6 g   **Fat** 6 g   **Protein** 12 g

6 servings
Per serving:
Energy 115 kcal/480 kJ
CHO 10 g (1 unit)
Fibre 4 g   **Fat** 4 g   **Protein** 8 g

Put the beans and soaking water in a pan, bring to the boil and boil for 10 minutes. Then lower the heat, cover and simmer for about 1½ hours or until the beans are soft, adding more water if necessary.

Drain the beans, return to the rinsed-out pan and mash well. Add the milk and onion and bring to the boil, stirring constantly. Simmer for 1 minute.

Remove the pan from the heat, then stir in the tomatoes, herbs, salt and pepper to taste. Stir in the egg yolks and leave to cool.

Beat the egg whites until just stiff, then fold into the bean sauce. Pour the mixture into a 1.5 litre (2½ pint) soufflé dish. Bake in a preheated moderate oven (180°C, 350°F, Gas Mark 4) for 1 hour or until the soufflé has risen and is lightly browned.

SPICY VEGETABLE CURRY

2 tablespoons polyunsaturated vegetable oil
1 teaspoon mustard seeds, crushed
1 × 5 cm (2 inch) piece root ginger, minced
2 garlic cloves, crushed
1 onion, minced
1 green chilli, seeded and minced
1½ teaspoons turmeric
1 tablespoon ground coriander
750 g / 1½–1¾ lb mixed vegetables
  (e.g. carrots, beans, aubergines, cauliflower)
salt

175 g / 6 oz coconut, puréed with 175 ml / 6 fl oz
  water
TO GARNISH
2 tablespoons chopped fresh coriander leaves
  (optional)

SERVES 4
Per serving:
Energy 260 kcal/1100 kJ
CHO 10 g (1 unit)
Fibre 11 g   **Fat** 23 g   **Protein** 4 g

Heat the oil in a large saucepan. Add the mustard seeds, ginger and garlic and fry for 30 seconds. Add the onion and green chilli and fry gently for 10 minutes, or until the onion is golden.

Stir in the turmeric and ground coriander and cook for 1 minute. Add the vegetables and stir to mix well with the fried

spices. Stir in the salt and coconut purée. If the mixture is too dry, add 1–2 tablespoons of water. Cover the pan and simmer for 30 minutes, or until the vegetables are tender when pierced with the point of a sharp knife. Turn into a warmed serving dish, sprinkle with the chopped coriander, if used, and serve with boiled rice.

PASTA WITH RATATOUILLE SAUCE

1 large onion, chopped
1 garlic clove, crushed
450 g / 1 lb courgettes, sliced
1 large aubergine, diced
1 green pepper, cored, seeded and diced
450 g / 1 lb tomatoes, chopped
1 tablespoon chopped oregano or basil
salt
freshly ground black pepper
450 g / 1 lb wholemeal pasta (e.g. noodles,
    spaghetti)
TO GARNISH
chopped parsley
grated Parmesan cheese to serve

SERVES 4–6
4 servings
Per serving:
Energy 390 kcal/1660 kJ
CHO 75 g (7.5 units)
Fibre 7 g   **Fat** 5 g   **Protein** 13 g

6 servings
Per serving:
Energy 260 kcal/1105 kJ
CHO 50 g (5 units)
Fibre 5 g   **Fat** 3 g   **Protein** 8 g

Put all the ingredients, except the pasta, into a large pan. Cover and cook gently for 30 minutes until the vegetables are tender and the juices have thickened slightly, stirring occasionally.

Meanwhile, cook the pasta in a large pan containing plenty of boiling salted water until just tender (about 5 minutes for freshly made pasta and 20 minutes for dried). Drain and pile into a warmed serving dish. Taste and adjust the seasoning of the sauce, then pour over the pasta. Sprinkle with the parsley and grated Parmesan cheese.

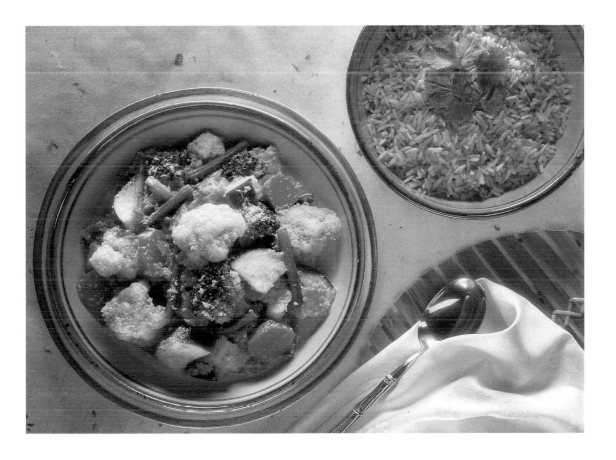

VEGETABLE TORTE

40 g/1½ oz polyunsaturated margarine
2 medium onions, finely chopped
50 g/2 oz carrots, peeled and thinly sliced
50 g/2 oz frozen peas
4 eggs
25 g/1 oz wholemeal flour
50 g/2 oz grated Parmesan cheese
3 tablespoons milk

2 tablespoons chopped parsley
salt and freshly ground black pepper

SERVES 4
Per serving:
Energy 250 kcal/1065 kJ
CHO 10 g (1 unit)
Fibre 2 g   **Fat** 19 g   **Protein** 14 g

Heat 25 g/1 oz of the margarine in a pan and fry the onions until just soft. Meanwhile cook the carrots and peas in a little salted water for 5 minutes only then drain them well.

Beat the eggs with the flour. Add the cheese to the eggs with the milk, vegetables, parsley and a little salt and pepper.

Grease the bottom and sides of an 18 cm (7 inch) soufflé dish or cake tin without a loose base, with the remaining margarine. Spoon in the egg mixture. Bake in a preheated moderate to moderately hot oven (180°–190°C, 350°–375°F, Gas Mark 4–5) for 30 minutes or until firm and golden in colour. Turn out and serve hot with vegetables or cold with salad.

BLACK-EYE PEA CASSEROLE

225 g/8 oz dried black-eye peas, soaked
    overnight in cold water
1 tablespoon polyunsaturated vegetable oil
1 large onion, chopped
2 garlic cloves, chopped
2 potatoes, peeled and sliced
2 large carrots, scraped and chopped
2 turnips, peeled and sliced
2 parsnips, peeled and sliced
2 celery sticks, chopped
1 tablespoon chopped fresh parsley
1 teaspoon dried thyme

1 teaspoon dried oregano
2 bay leaves
salt
freshly ground black pepper
2 tablespoons tomato purée
50 g/2 oz Cheddar cheese, grated (optional)

SERVES 4
Per serving:
Energy 180 kcal/755 kJ
CHO 20 g (2 units)
Fibre 5 g   **Fat** 9 g   **Protein** 8 g

Put the black-eye peas and their soaking water into a large saucepan. Bring to the boil, boil for 10 minutes, then cover and simmer gently for 20 minutes.

Meanwhile, heat the oil in a flameproof casserole, add the onion and garlic and fry until transparent. Stir in the potatoes, carrots, turnips, parsnips and celery. Cover tightly and cook over a gentle heat for 10 minutes, stirring occasionally to prevent the vegetables sticking to the pan.

Drain the black-eye peas, which should be almost tender, reserving their cooking liquid. Stir the drained peas into the cas-serole with the herbs and salt and pepper. Pour over 600 ml/1 pint of the reserved cooking liquid, adding more if necessary so that all the vegetables and peas are covered. Stir in the tomato purée. Cover tightly and transfer to a preheated moderate oven (180°C, 350°F, Gas Mark 4). Cook for 1½ hours.

Uncover the casserole and discard the bay leaves. Sprinkle with the grated cheese, if used. Cook without a lid for a further 10 minutes. This allows the juices in the pan to evaporate and thicken slightly, and for the cheese to melt.

COURGETTES WITH CORN

8 courgettes
1 tablespoon vegetable oil
1 onion, chopped
1 × 200 g (7 oz) can sweetcorn, drained

100 g/4 oz Cheddar cheese, grated
50 g/2 oz walnuts, chopped
salt
freshly ground black pepper

SERVES 6–8

6 servings **Per serving:**			**8 servings** **Per serving:**		
Energy 175 kcal/720 kJ			**Energy** 130 kcal/540 kJ		
CHO 10 g (1 unit)			**CHO** 5 g (0.5 units)		
Fibre 3 g	**Fat** 13 g	**Protein** 6 g	**Fibre** 2 g	**Fat** 10 g	**Protein** 4 g

Cut the courgettes in half lengthways, scoop out the flesh and chop finely. Blanch the shells in boiling water for 2 minutes and drain well.

Heat the oil in a pan and fry the onion and courgette flesh for 5 minutes until softened, then add the remaining ingredients and mix well. Arrange the courgette shells in a shallow ovenproof casserole, fill with the mixture, cover and bake in a preheated moderately hot oven (190°C, 375°F, Gas Mark 5) for 40 minutes.

SPICED RED BEANS

350 g/12 oz dried red kidney beans, soaked
    overnight in cold water
1 tablespoon polyunsaturated vegetable oil
1 large onion, chopped
225 g/8 oz mushrooms, chopped
25 g/1 oz desiccated coconut
2 tablespoons lemon juice
2 tablespoons grated lemon rind
salt
freshly ground black pepper
SAUCE
1 teaspoon ground cumin
½ teaspoon ground ginger
1 teaspoon ground coriander

1 teaspoon ground cardamom
4 tablespoons plain unsweetened yogurt
1 teaspoon tomato purée
1 tablespoon desiccated coconut
pinch of grated nutmeg
TO GARNISH
chopped parsley or coriander leaves

SERVES 4
Per serving:
Energy 340 kcal/1445 kJ
CHO 40 g (4 units)
Fibre 25 g **Fat** 10 g **Protein** 22 g

Put the beans and their soaking water into a large saucepan. Bring to the boil, boil for 10 minutes, then cover and simmer gently for 1–2 hours or until soft. Top up the water when necessary. Drain.

Heat the oil in another large saucepan, add the onion and fry until browned. Add the mushrooms and cook gently for a further 5 minutes, then stir in the beans.

Combine all the sauce ingredients in a bowl or blender and stir thoroughly or blend until smooth. Pour the sauce over the beans and vegetables.

Add the coconut and continue to cook gently for a few minutes. Pour the lemon juice over, add the lemon rind, salt and pepper to taste, and cook for a further 5–10 minutes, stirring constantly. Serve very hot, sprinkled with chopped parsley or coriander leaves.

LEEK PIE

PASTRY DOUGH
175 g / 6 oz wholemeal flour
pinch of salt
pinch of pepper
75 g / 3 oz polyunsaturated margarine, cut into
  small pieces
75 g / 3 oz mature Cheddar cheese, grated
2 tablespoons cold water
beaten egg or milk to glaze
FILLING
1 tablespoon polyunsaturated margarine
750 g / 1½–1¾ lb leeks, trimmed and sliced into
  1 cm / ½ inch rounds
25 g / 1 oz plain flour

300 ml / ½ pint stock or milk and water
1 tablespoon finely grated lemon rind
1 tablespoon lemon juice
½ teaspoon grated nutmeg
50 g / 2 oz hazelnuts
50 g / 2 oz seedless raisins
salt
freshly ground black pepper

SERVES 4
Per serving:
Energy 550 kcal / 2290 kJ
CHO 50 g (5 units)
Fibre 11 g **Fat** 31 g **Protein** 16 g

To make the pastry dough, put the flour, salt and pepper into a bowl, rub the margarine into the flour until the mixture resembles breadcrumbs, then stir in the cheese. Add the water and mix to a firm dough. Chill in the refrigerator until required for the pie.

To make the filling, melt the margarine in a pan. Add the leeks and fry gently for 5 minutes, stirring constantly until soft but not brown. Stir in the flour and cook for 1– 2 minutes. Gradually stir in the stock or milk and water. Bring to the boil, then lower the heat and simmer until the sauce is thick and smooth, stirring constantly. Add the remaining filling ingredients, simmer

for 2 minutes, then transfer to a 1 litre (1¾ pint) pie dish. Leave to cool.

Meanwhile, roll out the pastry dough on a lightly floured surface until 2.5 cm / 1 inch larger than the circumference of the pie dish. Cut a 1 cm / ½ inch strip from the edge, then press it on to the moistened rim of the dish. Moisten the strip, then cover the dish with the remaining pastry dough, pressing the edge firmly to seal. Trim and flute the edge, and decorate the top of the pie with the trimmings. Brush with beaten egg or milk. Bake in a preheated moderately hot oven (200°C, 400°F, Gas Mark 6) for 30 minutes or until the pastry is crisp and golden brown. Serve hot or cold.

WINTER CASSEROLE

1 aubergine, chopped
salt
1 tablespoon polyunsaturated vegetable oil
1 onion, chopped
1 garlic clove, chopped
4 carrots, scraped and chopped
2 celery sticks, chopped
2 parsnips, peeled and cut into 2.5 cm / 1 inch
  strips
225 g / 8 oz whole green or brown lentils, rinsed
900 ml / 1½ pints hot stock or water
1 bay leaf
1 sprig parsley

1 teaspoon dried marjoram
1 teaspoon tomato purée
freshly ground black pepper
225 g / 8 oz courgettes, thickly sliced
1 cauliflower, trimmed and cut into florets
TO GARNISH
chopped fresh parsley

SERVES 4
Per serving:
Energy 230 kcal / 1000 kJ
CHO 40 g (4 units)
Fibre 10 g **Fat** 3 g **Protein** 15 g

Put the aubergine into a colander. Sprinkle with salt and cover with a plate, weighted down. Leave for at least 30 minutes. Rinse the aubergine in cold water and drain on paper towels.

Heat the oil in a large, deep saucepan, add the onion and fry until transparent. Add the garlic and aubergine and fry for 5 minutes more. Stir in the carrots, celery, parsnips and lentils and pour over the hot stock or water. Bring to the boil, then boil for 10 minutes, skimming if necessary.

Add the bay leaf, parsley, marjoram, tomato purée, salt and pepper. Cover tightly and simmer very gently for 35 minutes, stirring occasionally so that the lentils don't stick to the bottom of the pan.

Add the courgettes and cauliflower with a little more hot stock or water if there is not enough liquid in the pan. Cover tightly again and simmer gently for a further 15 minutes or until the vegetables are tender and the liquid has been absorbed. Should there be too much liquid, cook uncovered for a few minutes.

Taste and adjust the seasoning, and discard the bay leaf, then transfer the vegetable mixture to a warmed serving dish. Sprinkle with parsley and serve with a green salad.

CUCUMBER MOUSSE WITH HAM

½ packet unsweetened lemon jelly
150 ml / ¼ pint boiling water
1 cucumber
salt and freshly ground black pepper
2 × 225 g (8 oz) cartons cottage cheese

150 ml / ¼ pint plain unsweetened yogurt
6 tablespoons cold water
15 g / ½ oz powdered gelatine
lemon juice or wine vinegar
8 slices cooked ham, rolled

SERVES 4–6

4 servings Per serving:			**6 servings** Per serving:		
Energy 165 kcal/685 kJ			**Energy** 110 kcal/460 kJ		
CHO 5 g (0.5 units)			**CHO** 0 g (0 units)		
Fibre 0 g	**Fat** 6 g	**Protein** 22 g	**Fibre** 0 g	**Fat** 4 g	**Protein** 14 g

Dissolve the jelly in the boiling water and allow to cool. Make a layer of the jelly on the bottom of a 900 ml (1½ pint) ring mould. Thinly slice quarter of the unpeeled cucumber, quarter the slices and arrange in the jelly. Allow to set.

Peel the remaining cucumber, cut in half lengthways and remove the seeds. Chop the flesh and place in a colander. Sprinkle with salt and leave for 1 hour to draw the juices. Rinse and drain well, then pat dry with absorbent kitchen paper.

Press the cottage cheese through a fine sieve into a mixing bowl. Stir in the plain yogurt.

Place the cold water in a small saucepan. Sprinkle over the gelatine. Allow to soak for a few minutes, then stir over a low heat until the gelatine has dissolved. Cool slightly, then stir into the cottage cheese mixture. Add salt, pepper and lemon juice or wine vinegar to taste. Fold in the chopped cucumber. When the mixture begins to set, pour into the ring mould on top of the jelly mixture. Chill until set.

To turn out of the mould, dip into hot water for 15 seconds, then invert quickly on to a serving dish. Arrange the rolled slices of ham in the centre.

Desserts

APPLE MOUSSE

450 g / 1 lb cooking apples, cored and sliced
3 tablespoons water
300 ml / ½ pint unsweetened grapefruit juice
3 teaspoons powdered gelatine
few drops artificial sweetener
1 egg white
pinch of nutmeg

SERVES 4
Per serving:
Energy 80 kcal / 350 kJ
CHO 20 g (2 units)
Fibre 2 g   **Fat** 0 g   **Protein** 1 g

Simmer the apples (reserving a few slices for decoration) with the water until tender. Heat a little of the grapefruit juice and dissolve the gelatine in it. When the apples have cooled slightly, sieve or purée in a blender with the dissolved gelatine. Whisk in the remaining grapefruit juice with sweetener to taste. Place the mixture in an ice tray and freeze until beginning to set.

Whisk the egg white until stiff. Take out the apple purée and whisk again until frothy, adding the nutmeg. Fold in the egg white and freeze until stiff but not solid. Spoon into individual serving dishes and decorate with slices of apple.

PASSION FRUIT PAVLOVA

3 large egg whites
1 teaspoon cream of tartar
3 tablespoons dry skimmed milk
6 saccharin tablets, crushed
4 passion fruit
2 oranges, peeled and segmented
TO DECORATE
mint sprigs

SERVES 4
Per serving:
Energy 70 kcal / 300 kJ
CHO 11 g (1 unit)
Fibre 6 g   **Fat** 0 g   **Protein** 6 g

Whisk the egg whites lightly, sprinkle in the cream of tartar and continue whisking until the mixture forms peaks. Add the milk and saccharin a little at a time, until the peaks are stiff.

Draw a circle round a 20 cm (8 inch) plate on a piece of non-stick silicone paper. Place on a baking sheet and spread the meringue mixture smoothly in the circle. Cook in a preheated cool oven (150°C, 300°F, Gas Mark 2) for about 30 minutes.

Cool, loosen the meringue carefully with a palette knife and lift on to a serving dish. Scoop out the centres of the passion fruit and pile on top of the meringue, with orange segments. Decorate with mint.

CLOCKWISE FROM THE TOP: PASSION FRUIT PAVLOVA; APPLE MOUSSE; LEMON AND BLACKCURRANT DESSERT (P. 68)

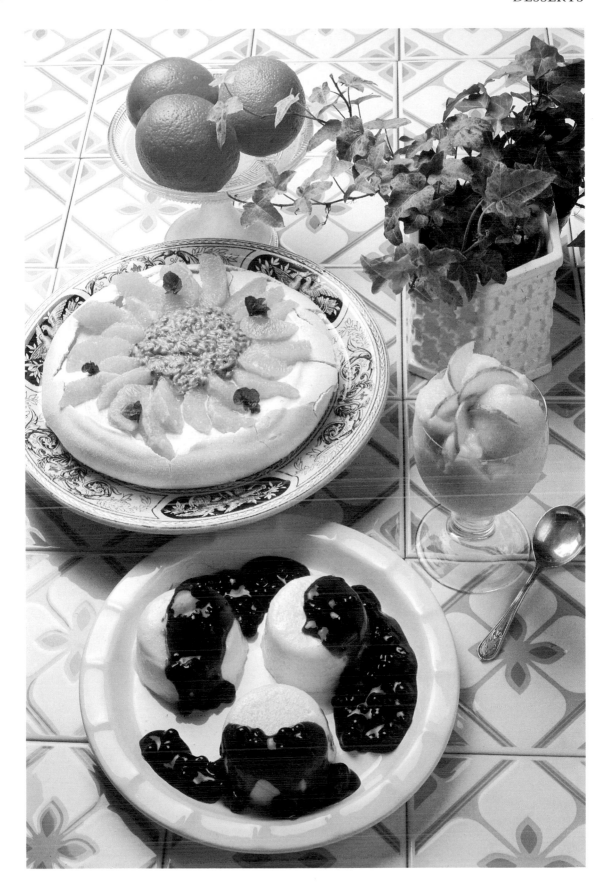

LEMON AND BLACKCURRANT DESSERT

½ × 150 g (5 oz) tablet unsweetened lemon jelly
65 ml / 2½ fl oz boiling water
¼ teaspoon finely grated lemon rind
1 tablespoon lemon juice
1 egg white
100 g / 4 oz fresh blackcurrants
1½ teaspoons cornflour
2 tablespoons cold water

few drops vanilla essence
liquid sweetener

SERVES 4
Per serving:
Energy 35 kcal / 145 kJ
CHO 7 g (0.5 units)
Fibre 1 g **Fat** 0 g **Protein** 1 g

Dissolve the lemon jelly in a large bowl with the boiling water. Make up to 250 ml/8 fl oz with cold water. Stir in the lemon rind and juice. Chill until almost set. Add the egg white to the jelly mixture and beat with an electric whisk until light and fluffy – about 2 minutes. Pour into a mould or four ramekin dishes and chill until firm.

Meanwhile crush a third of the blackcurrants in a saucepan. Blend together the cornflour and cold water and add to the crushed blackcurrants. Cook over a medium heat, stirring constantly, until the mixture is thick and bubbly. Remove from heat and stir in remaining blackcurrants and vanilla essence. Sweeten to taste.

To serve, unmould the lemon jelly into a dish and spoon over the blackcurrant sauce. *Illustrated on page 67.*

ORANGE SORBET

2 tablespoons lemon juice
1 teaspoon artificial sweetener
2 tablespoons grated orange rind
1 × 175 g (6 fl oz) can unsweetened concentrated orange juice
1 egg white, stiffly beaten
TO DECORATE
orange slices

SERVES 4
Per serving:
Energy 20 kcal / 95 kJ
CHO 0 g (0 units)
Fibre 0 g **Fat** 0 g **Protein** 0 g

Mix together the lemon juice and sweetener and make up to 300 ml/½ pint with water. Add the orange rind and orange juice and pour into an ice tray. Freeze until just firm. Turn out into a mixing bowl and mash with a fork until the crystals are broken down. Fold the beaten egg white into the mixture, using a metal spoon. Return to the ice tray and freeze until firm.

Soften slightly in the refrigerator for about 20 minutes before serving. Decorate with twists of orange.

ORANGE SURPRISE

4 oranges
1 banana, peeled and finely chopped
1 dessert apple, unpeeled and finely chopped
artificial sweetener

SERVES 4
Per serving:
Energy 80 kcal / 340 kJ
CHO 20 g (2 units)
Fibre 4 g **Fat** 0 g **Protein** 1 g

Cut a thin slice from the base of each orange so that they will stand firmly. Cut off the tops so that the flesh is just showing and scoop out all the flesh with a teaspoon, discarding any pips. Add the chopped banana and apple to the orange flesh, with sweetener to taste. Pile back into the orange shells and chill in the refrigerator before serving.

RHUBARB AND GINGER SOUFFLÉ

500 g / 1¼ lb rhubarb, trimmed and cut into
    2.5 cm / 1 inch pieces
50 g / 2 oz polyunsaturated margarine
50 g / 2 oz wholemeal breadcrumbs
200 ml / ⅓ pint semi-skimmed milk
3 eggs, separated
½ teaspoon ground ginger
artificial sweetener equivalent to 25 g / 1 oz
    sugar

SERVES 4
Per serving:
Energy 215 kcal / 890 kJ
CHO 10 g (1 unit)
Fibre 3 g   **Fat** 16 g   **Protein** 9 g

Place the rhubarb in a saucepan and add a few drops of water. Cook gently until the fruit is soft. Strain off most of the liquid.

Place the margarine, breadcrumbs and milk in a saucepan. Heat, whisking for 2–3 minutes until smooth. Cool slightly, then beat in the egg yolks, ginger, rhubarb and sweetener. Whisk the egg whites until stiff and fold into the mixture. Turn into a greased 15 cm (6 inch) soufflé dish. Cook in a moderately hot oven (200°C, 400°F, Gas Mark 6) for 35–40 minutes until well risen. Serve immediately.

APRICOT SYLLABUB

225 g / 8 oz dried apricots, soaked overnight in
    600 ml / 1 pint water
1 tablespoon finely grated lemon rind
3 tablespoons lemon juice
150 ml / ¼ pint plain unsweetened yogurt
2 tablespoons Grand Marnier
artificial sweetener equivalent to 50 g / 2 oz
    sugar
2 egg whites

TO DECORATE
lemon twists or chopped nuts

SERVES 6
Per serving:
Energy 85 kcal / 360 kJ
CHO 18 g (2 units)
Fibre 9 g   **Fat** 0 g   **Protein** 4 g

Put the apricots and soaking liquid into a saucepan with the lemon rind and juice and bring to the boil. Lower the heat, cover and simmer for 20–30 minutes until the apricots are soft, adding more water if necessary. Work the mixture to a smooth purée in a blender or food processor, then transfer to a bowl and leave to cool.

Stir the yogurt, Grand Marnier and sweetener into the purée, blending well. Beat the egg whites until just stiff, then fold into the mixture, using a metal spoon. Spoon into a bowl or six individual dishes and refrigerate for at least 1 hour before serving. Decorate with lemon twists or chopped nuts.

GRAPE-STUFFED APPLES

4 medium cooking apples, washed and cored
150 ml / ¼ pint dry cider
artificial sweetener
100 g / 4 oz grapes, washed, halved and seeded
4 small bunches grapes, washed
egg white
25 g / 1 oz desiccated coconut

SERVES 4
Per serving:
Energy 115 kcal / 490 kJ
CHO 18 g (2 units)
Fibre 4 g **Fat** 3 g **Protein** 0 g

Put the apples into a shallow ovenproof dish. Mix the cider with sweetener – allow for the tartness of the apples. Pack the grapes into the centre of each apple and pour over the cider mixture. Cover with foil and bake in a preheated moderate oven (180°C, 350°F, Gas Mark 4) for 45 minutes.

Meanwhile dip each small bunch of grapes in a little egg white and roll in the coconut. Allow to dry. Decorate each baked apple with a bunch of the frosted grapes.

STRAWBERRY SOUFFLÉ

25 g / 1 oz powdered gelatine
400 ml / 14 fl oz boiling water
600 ml / 1 pint low-calorie orange squash,
  undiluted
2 teaspoons finely grated lemon rind
artificial sweetener
450 g / 1 lb fresh strawberries, hulled and sliced

SERVES 4
Per serving:
Energy 55 kcal / 230 kJ
CHO 13 g (1 unit)
Fibre 2 g **Fat** 0 g **Protein** 0 g

Dissolve the gelatine in the boiling water, then stir in the orange squash and lemon rind. Make up to 1.2 litres/2 pints with cold water. Sweeten to taste with the sweetener. Leave to chill until just beginning to set. Whisk until light and foamy and spoon into shallow dessert dishes. Chill until firm and set. Just before serving top with the sliced strawberries.

LEFT: STRAWBERRY SOUFFLÉ; RIGHT: GRAPE-STUFFED APPLES

GRAPE JELLY

15 g / ½ oz powdered gelatine
150 ml / ¼ pint boiling water
450 ml / ¾ pint unsweetened grape juice
225 g / 8 oz green grapes, washed, peeled and
    seeded
225 g / 8 oz cottage cheese
2 × 150 ml / ¼ pint cartons plain unsweetened
    yogurt

SERVES 6
Per serving:
Energy 110 kcal / 470 kJ
CHO 16 g (1.5 units)
Fibre 0 g   **Fat** 1 g   **Protein** 8 g

Dissolve the gelatine in the boiling water and add the grape juice. Pour into six tall glasses. Divide the grapes between the glasses and leave tilted in a cool place to set. Blend or sieve the cottage cheese until smooth. Fold in the yogurt and top up the glasses.

Chill the jelly before serving.

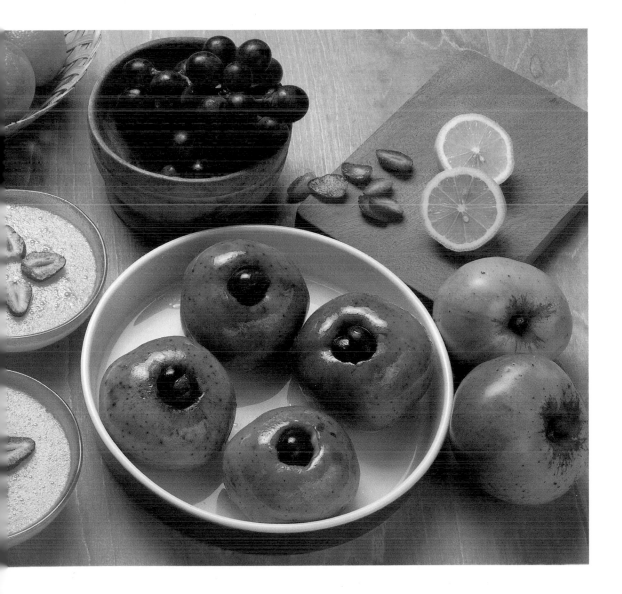

APRICOT SOUFFLÉ

1 × 225 g (8 oz) can apricots in natural juice,
  drained
2 eggs, separated
artificial sweetener
15 g/½ oz powdered gelatine
1 tablespoon lemon juice
1 × 175 ml (6 fl oz) can evaporated milk

SERVES 4
Per serving:
Energy 125 kcal/520 kJ
CHO 10 g (1 unit)
Fibre 0 g   **Fat** 7 g   **Protein** 7 g

Reserve 1–2 apricots for decoration and purée the remainder in a blender or food processor or by rubbing through a sieve.

Place the apricot purée in a heavy saucepan with the egg yolks and cook over a low heat, stirring lightly, until thickened. Remove from the heat and stir in the sweetener to taste. Sprinkle the gelatine over and stir to dissolve. Add the lemon juice and cool until beginning to thicken.

Whip the evaporated milk until it holds its shape, then fold in the apricot mixture. Turn into four individual glasses and chill. Decorate the soufflés with slices of the reserved apricots.

COMPÔTE

150 ml/¼ pint water
2–3 strips lemon rind
3–4 tablespoons lemon juice
4 tablespoons orange juice
1 large cooking apple, peeled, cored and sliced
100 g/4 oz blackberries
100 g/4 oz damsons, stoned
100 g/4 oz black plums, stoned
100 g/4 oz golden plums, stoned

artificial sweetener equivalent to 50 g/2 oz
  sugar

SERVES 4
Per serving:
Energy 55 kcal/230 kJ
CHO 13 g (1 unit)
Fibre 5 g   **Fat** 0 g   **Protein** 1 g

Put the water in a large, heavy pan. Add the lemon rind, lemon juice and orange juice. Bring to the boil, stirring. Add the apple, blackberries, damsons, plums and sweetener. Simmer gently until the fruit is cooked. Remove the lemon rind and serve either hot or cold.

FRESH FRUIT SALAD

300 ml/½ pint water
2 tablespoons lemon juice
1–2 tablespoons Cointreau
2 oranges, peeled and segmented
2 bananas, peeled and thickly sliced
2 dessert apples, washed and sliced
50 g/2 oz black grapes, seeded
50 g/2 oz green grapes, seeded
1 pear, sliced

SERVES 4
Per serving:
Energy 125 kcal/535 kJ
CHO 30 g (3 units)
Fibre 5 g   **Fat** 0 g   **Protein** 2 g

When available, fruits such as melon, strawberries or raspberries can be added without appreciably altering the calorie or carbohydrate content of this recipe.

Mix together the water, lemon juice and Cointreau. Place the prepared fruits in a large bowl and pour the liquid over. Mix well and leave to stand for 2–3 hours. Transfer to a serving bowl. This salad can be served with plain unsweetened yogurt.

BRAMBLE MOUSSE

450 g / 1 lb blackberries
225 g / 8 oz cooking apples, peeled, cored and sliced
2 tablespoons orange juice
2 tablespoons finely grated orange rind
15 g / ½ oz powdered gelatine

2 tablespoons water
150 ml / ¼ pint plain unsweetened yogurt
artificial sweetener equivalent to 40 g / 1½ oz sugar
2 egg whites

SERVES 4–6

4 servings Per serving:			**6 servings** Per serving:		
Energy 80 kcal / 340 kJ			**Energy** 50 kcal / 225 kJ		
CHO 15 g (1.5 units)			**CHO** 10 g (1 unit)		
Fibre 9 g	**Fat** 0 g	**Protein** 4 g	**Fibre** 6 g	**Fat** 0 g	**Protein** 2 g

Put the blackberries in a pan, reserving a few for decoration. Add the apples, orange juice and rind. Cover and heat gently for 10–15 minutes until the fruit is soft, stirring occasionally. Rub the blackberries through a sieve into a bowl.

Sprinkle the gelatine over the water in a small cup. Stand the cup in a pan of hot water and stir until the gelatine has dissolved. Stir the gelatine into the fruit purée with the yogurt and sweetener and mix well. Leave the purée mixture in a cool place until thick and just beginning to set.

Beat the egg whites until just stiff, then fold into the mousse. Transfer to a large serving bowl or individual dishes or glasses. Chill in the refrigerator until set, then decorate with the reserved blackberries. Serve chilled.

GRAPES AND ORANGES

6 oranges, peel and pith removed
2 tablespoons lemon juice
1 tablespoon grated lemon rind
few drops vanilla essence
225 g / 8 oz black grapes, seeded

SERVES 4
Per serving:
Energy 80 kcal / 350 kJ
CHO 20 g (2 units)
Fibre 3 g   **Fat** 0 g   **Protein** 1 g

Slice the oranges across thinly, taking care to keep all the juice. Put this juice in a small pan, together with the lemon juice. Add the lemon rind and vanilla essence. Bring to the boil, and cook quickly until well reduced.

Allow to cool, then pour over the oranges, discarding the lemon rind. Add the grapes and chill before serving.

RHUBARB FOOL

450 g / 1 lb rhubarb, washed, trimmed and cut
into 5 cm / 2 inch lengths
3 tablespoons cold water
2 tablespoons lemon juice
1 tablespoon finely grated lemon rind
artificial sweetener
2 egg yolks
150 ml / ¼ pint plain unsweetened yogurt

SERVES 4
Per serving:

Energy	70 kcal / 280 kJ		
CHO	0 g (0 units)		
Fibre	2 g	**Fat** 4 g	**Protein** 4 g

Put the rhubarb into a saucepan with the water, lemon juice, lemon rind and sweetener to taste. Simmer gently until tender. Purée in a blender or sieve.

When cool, beat in the egg yolks and fold in the yogurt so that the fool is streaked with threads of rhubarb. Spoon into sundae dishes and chill.

LEFT: RHUBARB FOOL; RIGHT: ORANGE CHEESE

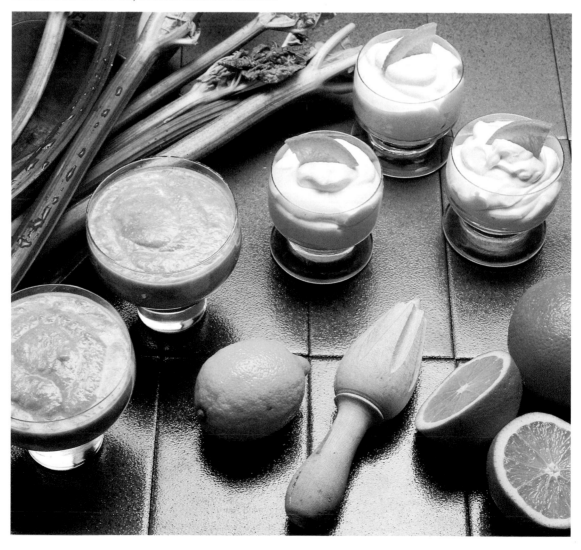

ORANGE CHEESE

3 tablespoons orange juice
4 teaspoons lemon juice
4 teaspoons powdered gelatine
350 g / 12 oz cottage cheese
6 tablespoons buttermilk
artificial sweetener
TO DECORATE
1 orange, thinly sliced

SERVES 4
Per serving:
Energy 100 kcal / 415 kJ
CHO   0 g (0 units)
Fibre   0 g   **Fat** 3 g   **Protein** 12 g

Put the orange and lemon juices in a small bowl and sprinkle the gelatine over the top. Stand over a bowl of hot, but not boiling, water to dissolve the gelatine, then put into a blender with the cottage cheese and buttermilk and blend until smooth. Add sweetener to taste. Divide the mixture between four dessert glasses and decorate with quartered slices of orange.

PEACH AND RASPBERRY CHEESECAKE

75 g / 3 oz polyunsaturated margarine
175 g / 6 oz digestive biscuits, crushed
FILLING
350 g / 12 oz cottage cheese, sieved
150 ml / ¼ pint plain unsweetened yogurt
artificial sweetener equivalent to 50 g / 2 oz
   sugar
1 tablespoon finely grated lemon rind

2 tablespoons lemon juice
15 g / ½ oz powdered gelatine
2 tablespoons water
2 egg whites
TOPPING
2 large peaches, stoned and sliced
225 g / 8 oz raspberries

SERVES 6–8
6 servings
Per serving:
Energy 320 kcal / 1330 kJ
CHO   25 g (2.5 units)
Fibre   4 g   **Fat** 18 g   **Protein** 13 g

8 servings
Per serving:
Energy 240 kcal / 995 kJ
CHO   20 g (2 units)
Fibre   3 g   **Fat** 14 g   **Protein** 9 g

To make the crust, melt the margarine in a pan, then stir in the biscuits. Spoon the mixture into a lightly greased 18–20 cm (7–8 inch) loose-bottomed cake tin, spread evenly and press down with the back of a spoon. Chill in the refrigerator.

Meanwhile, make the filling, put the cottage cheese in a bowl with the yogurt, sweetener, lemon rind and juice, reserving 1 tablespoon of lemon juice for the topping. Beat well. Sprinkle the gelatine over the water in a small cup. Stand the cup in a pan of hot water and stir until the gelatine has dissolved. Fold the gelatine into the cheese mixture.

Beat the egg whites until stiff, then fold into the cheese mixture. Pour on top of the crust in the tin and level the surface. Chill in the refrigerator until set.

To serve, run a knife around the edge of the cheesecake, then remove from the tin. Brush the cut surfaces of the sliced peaches with the reserved lemon juice and arrange on top of the cheesecake with the raspberries. Serve chilled.

International Dishes

CHINESE SALAD

275 g/10 oz fresh bean-sprouts, rinsed and
   thoroughly dried
100 g/4 oz button mushrooms, thinly sliced
1 bunch spring onions, chopped
1 chicken portion (about 175 g/6 oz), cooked
   and shredded
1 banana, peeled and sliced
1 × 200 g (7 oz) can unsweetened peach slices,
   drained and chopped
4 celery sticks, chopped
25 g/1 oz cashew nuts
DRESSING
150 ml/¼ pint plain unsweetened yogurt

2 tablespoons soy sauce
1 tablespoon wine vinegar
salt
freshly ground black pepper
TO GARNISH
celery leaves

SERVES 4
Per serving:
Energy 180 kcal/755 kJ
CHO 18 g (2 units)
Fibre 7 g   **Fat** 5 g   **Protein** 16 g

Put the bean-sprouts into a bowl and add the other ingredients.

Put the dressing ingredients into a screw-topped jar and shake well. Pour the dressing over the salad and toss well. Garnish with the celery leaves.

AMERICAN MOULD

1 lime-flavoured, sugar-free jelly
150 ml/¼ pint boiling water
150 ml/¼ pint dry cider
2 celery sticks, chopped
1 green-skinned apple, unpeeled, quartered,
   cored and thinly sliced
¼ cucumber, thinly sliced
FILLING
225 g/8 oz low-fat soft cheese
4 tablespoons semi-skimmed milk
2–3 tablespoons fresh chives, chopped

50 g/3 oz walnuts, chopped
TO GARNISH
chopped chives
chopped walnuts

SERVES 4–6
Per serving:
Energy 105 kcal/440 kJ
CHO 5 g (0.5 units)
Fibre 1 g   **Fat** 6 g   **Protein** 6 g

Dissolve the jelly in the boiling water. Stir in the cider with enough cold water or ice cubes to make the liquid up to 450 ml/¾ pint. Pour a third of the liquid into a 1 litre (1¾ pint) ring mould and scatter in the chopped celery. Chill until set. Keep the remaining jelly liquid.

Pour half the remaining jelly on top and arrange the apple slices around the ring. Chill again until set. Keep the remaining jelly liquid.

Pour in the remaining jelly, then arrange the cucumber on top of the apple, ensuring that all the slices are submerged in jelly. Chill the ring for 2 hours or until required.

For the filling, beat the cheese with the milk until evenly blended. Stir in the chives and walnuts.

To serve, dip the mould in hot water for 20 seconds, then invert it on to a plate. Fill the centre with the cheese mixture and garnish with a few extra chopped chives and walnuts. *Illustrated on page 38.*

GREEK MUSHROOMS AND LEEKS

1 tablespoon polyunsaturated vegetable oil
1 large onion, sliced
1 large garlic clove, crushed
1 celery stick, sliced
225 g/8 oz leeks, sliced
150 ml/¼ pint dry white wine
225 g/8 oz tomatoes, quartered and seeds removed
salt
freshly ground black pepper
1 tablespoon chopped parsley
1 tablespoon dried thyme
1 bay leaf
225 g/8 oz button mushrooms
TO GARNISH
2 tablespoons chopped parsley

SERVES 4
Per serving:
Energy 85 kcal/350 kJ
CHO 7 g (1 unit)
Fibre 3 g **Fat** 2 g **Protein** 2 g

Heat the oil in a large pan and add the onion, garlic, celery and leeks. Cook gently for 5 minutes without browning. Add the wine, tomatoes, salt, pepper and herbs, and bring to the boil. Add the mushrooms and simmer gently for 10 minutes.

Leave to cool, then pour into a serving dish and chill. Serve cold, sprinkled with chopped parsley.

GAZPACHO

450 g/1 lb ripe juicy tomatoes, skinned
1 large onion, chopped
1 small green pepper, cored, seeded and chopped
1 garlic clove, finely chopped
1 tablespoon wine vinegar
1 tablespoon polyunsaturated vegetable oil
2 tablespoons lemon juice
150 ml/¼ pint tomato juice
salt and freshly ground black pepper
TO GARNISH
½ cucumber, peeled and diced

SERVES 4
Per serving:
Energy 50 kcal/220 kJ
CHO 6 g (0.5 units)
Fibre 2 g **Fat** 2 g **Protein** 1 g

Purée the tomatoes, onion, green pepper, garlic, vinegar and oil in a blender, or rub through a fine sieve. Turn into a bowl, add the lemon juice and tomato juice, season to taste and chill thoroughly in the refrigerator. Serve the Gazpacho sprinkled with the diced cucumber.

MINESTRONE

1 tablespoon polyunsaturated vegetable oil
1 onion, finely chopped
1 garlic clove, crushed
25 g/1 oz lean bacon, rinded and diced
75 g/3 oz haricot beans, soaked overnight in
    900 ml/1½ pints stock
salt and freshly ground black pepper
2 tablespoons finely chopped celery
1 large carrot, scrubbed and diced
225 g/8 oz cabbage, finely shredded

50 g/2 oz wholemeal macaroni
TO GARNISH
25 g/1 oz grated Parmesan cheese
1 tablespoon finely chopped parsley

SERVES 4
Per serving:
Energy 210 kcal/880 kJ
CHO   20 g (2 units)
Fibre   8 g   **Fat** 8 g   **Protein** 11 g

Heat the oil in a saucepan and toss the onion in it, with the garlic and bacon. Add the haricot beans and stock, salt and pepper. Simmer gently for about 1½ hours. Add all remaining vegetables except the cabbage and cook for a further 20 minutes, adding a little more stock if needed. Add the cabbage and macaroni and cook until both are just tender. Adjust the seasoning. Serve sprinkled with Parmesan cheese and garnished with chopped parsley.

YUGOSLAVIAN SPINACH SOUP

1 tablespoon polyunsaturated vegetable oil
1 medium onion, finely chopped
2 tablespoons ground almonds
100 g/4 oz brown rice
1 litre/1¾ pints chicken stock
450 g/1 lb spinach, coarsely shredded

salt
freshly ground black pepper
1–2 tablespoons chopped dill
300 ml/½ pint plain unsweetened yogurt
2–3 slices wholemeal bread
75 g/3 oz cottage cheese

SERVES 4–6

4 servings
Per serving:
Energy 280 kcal/1180 kJ
CHO   35 g (3.5 units)
Fibre   3 g   **Fat** 9 g   **Protein** 14 g

6 servings
Per serving:
Energy 190 kcal/785 kJ
CHO   25 g (2.5 units)
Fibre   2 g   **Fat** 6 g   **Protein** 9 g

Heat the oil in a large saucepan, fry the onion until nearly tender, then add the ground almonds and cook until a delicate brown colour. Stir in the rice and blend with the onion and almonds. Pour in the stock, bring to the boil, then add the spinach. Simmer steadily for 15–20 minutes or until the rice is tender. Add salt and pepper, the dill and half the yogurt. Heat gently.

Meanwhile, toast the bread, cut into triangles and spread with the cheese. Spoon the soup into individual soup cups and top with the remaining yogurt; serve with the cheese-spread toast.

VARIATION
The cheese can be varied. In Yugoslavia sheep's cheese is used. If using frozen leaf or chopped spinach, allow 350 g/12 oz only. This does not need as much cooking as fresh spinach so add after cooking the rice for about 10 minutes.

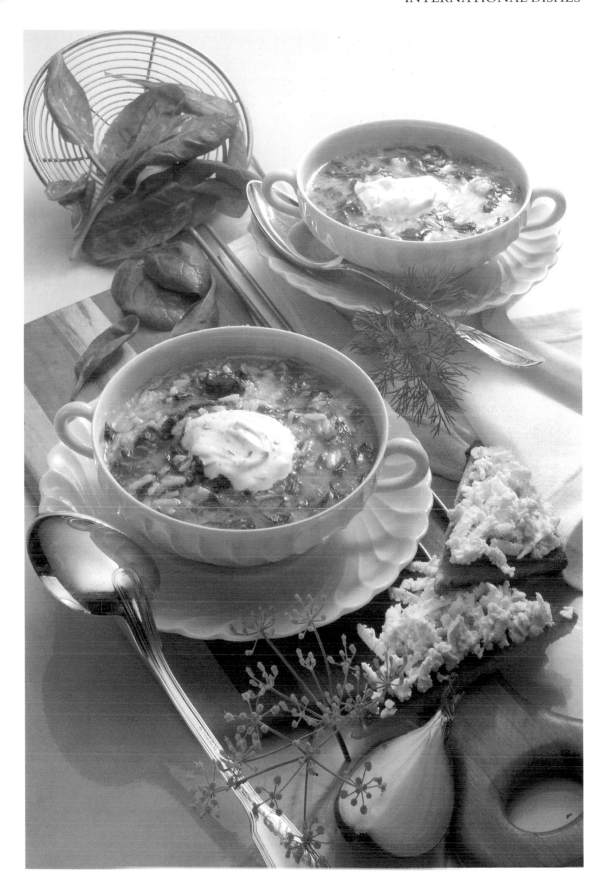

BOUILLABAISSE

1 tablespoon polyunsaturated vegetable oil
1 large onion, sliced
1 garlic clove, crushed
2 × 400 g/14 oz cans tomatoes
300 ml/½ pint fish stock
2 tablespoons chopped parsley
1 bouquet garni
salt
freshly ground black pepper
450 g/1 lb monkfish, diced
750 g/1½ lb red fish, skinned and filleted

350 g/12 oz coley fillets, skinned and diced
4 × 175 g (6 oz) plaice fillets, skinned and cut
   into strips
TO GARNISH
parsley

SERVES 8
Per serving:
Energy 305 kcal/1275 kJ
CHO 0 g (0 units)
Fibre 1 g   **Fat** 15 g   **Protein** 39 g

Any fish can be used to make bouillabaisse, but it is important to cook the firmer fish first, then to add the flakier ones. Shellfish, such as prawns, lobster pieces, mussels or clams, can also be added.

Heat the oil in a large pan and cook the onion and garlic gently for 5 minutes. Add the tomatoes and their juice, the stock, parsley, bouquet garni, salt and pepper to taste. Bring to the boil, then simmer for 10 minutes. Add the monkfish and red fish and cook for 5 minutes. Stir in the coley and cook for a further 5 minutes. Finally, add the plaice and simmer for 5–10 minutes or until all the fish is cooked. Remove the bouquet garni and adjust the seasoning. Pour the soup into a tureen and sprinkle with chopped parsley. Serve with warm wholemeal bread.

GREEK VEGETABLE SOUP

450 ml/¾ pint beef stock
100 g/4 oz mixed vegetables, chopped
1 egg yolk
300 ml/½ pint plain unsweetened yogurt

salt and freshly ground black pepper
TO GARNISH
1 tablespoon chopped mint leaves
1 tablespoon finely grated lemon rind

SERVES 4–6

4 servings
Per serving:
Energy 75 kcal/385 kJ
CHO 5 g (0.5 units)
Fibre 0 g   **Fat** 3 g   **Protein** 5 g

6 servings
Per serving:
Energy 50 kcal/260 kJ
CHO 0 g (0 units)
Fibre 0 g   **Fat** 2 g   **Protein** 3 g

Put the stock in a pan and bring to the boil. Add the vegetables, then lower the heat, cover and simmer for 10 minutes or until just tender.

Meanwhile, put the egg yolk in a bowl and whisk in the yogurt. Stir in 6 tablespoons of the hot liquid and mix well. Add to the soup in the pan, stirring constantly. Heat through gently without boiling. Season with salt and pepper to taste.

Pour into four individual serving bowls, garnish with chopped mint and lemon rind and serve hot.

ITALIAN BEAN SOUP

225 g/8 oz dried white beans (haricot, butter
    beans, etc), soaked overnight in 600 ml/1
    pint water
stock or water
1 large onion, chopped
1 garlic clove, crushed (optional)
1 celery stick, sliced
1 large carrot, peeled and sliced

4 tomatoes, skinned and chopped
1 tablespoon finely grated lemon rind
1 tablespoon lemon juice
1 bay leaf
salt
freshly ground black pepper
TO GARNISH
2 tablespoons chopped parsley (optional)

SERVES 4–6

4 servings
Per serving:
Energy 200 kcal/845 kJ
CHO 35 g (3.5 units)
Fibre 17 g **Fat** 0 g **Protein** 14 g

6 servings
Per serving:
Energy 130 kcal/560 kJ
CHO 25 g (2.5 units)
Fibre 11 g **Fat** 0 g **Protein** 9 g

Drain the beans, reserving the soaking liquid. Make this up to 1.2 litres/2 pints with stock or more water.

Place the beans and liquid in a large pan and add the remaining ingredients. Bring to the boil, then lower the heat, cover and simmer for 1–1½ hours or until the beans are tender, adding more water if necessary.

Discard the bay leaf.

Transfer about half the beans and some of the liquid to a blender and purée until smooth. Return the purée to the soup and bring to the boil, stirring constantly. Taste and adjust the seasoning, and add more liquid if the soup is too thick. Sprinkle with parsley if liked and serve hot.

RATATOUILLE

2 tablespoons polyunsaturated vegetable oil
2 medium onions, sliced
2 garlic cloves, crushed
2 medium aubergines, chopped
1 green pepper, cored, seeded and chopped
1 red pepper, cored, seeded and chopped
1 chilli, seeded and chopped
3 courgettes, thinly sliced
750 g/1½–1¾ lb tomatoes, chopped
1 teaspoon salt
freshly ground black pepper
1 teaspoon paprika

dash of Tabasco sauce
1 teaspoon chopped fresh basil
1 teaspoon chopped fresh chives
1 tablespoon tomato purée
TO GARNISH
50 g/2 oz Parmesan cheese

SERVES 8
Per serving:
Energy 80 kcal/320 kJ
CHO 0 g (0 units)
Fibre 2 g **Fat** 5 g **Protein** 4 g

Heat the oil in a large heavy frying pan and cook the onions and garlic together for about 5 minutes or until just translucent. Add the aubergines, peppers, chilli and courgettes. Stir thoroughly and cook together for about 5 minutes. Add the remaining ingredients. Bring to the boil, then reduce the heat and simmer slowly for 45 minutes, stirring occasionally.

Serve as a starter, sprinkled with the grated Parmesan.

JAPANESE STEAMED WHOLE FISH

2 Chinese dried mushrooms, soaked in tepid
    water for 20 minutes
450 g/1 lb sea bass or perch, scaled and cleaned
2 slices ginger root, peeled and finely shredded
2 spring onions, finely shredded
50 g/2 oz cooked ham, finely shredded
50 g/2 oz bamboo shoots, finely shredded
3 tablespoons dry sherry

3 tablespoons soy sauce
1 teaspoon salt

SERVES 4
Per serving:
Energy 200 kcal/830 kJ
CHO   4 g (0.5 units)
Fibre   0 g   **Fat** 5 g   **Protein** 29 g

Squeeze the mushrooms dry and discard the stalks.

Slash both sides of the fish diagonally as deep as the bone at intervals of about 1 cm/ ½ inch. This prevents the skin from bursting in cooking, allows the heat to penetrate more quickly and helps to diffuse the flavour of the seasonings and sauce. Dry the fish thoroughly with paper towels,

then place it on a plate.

Arrange the ginger root, spring onions, ham, mushrooms and bamboo shoots on top of the fish. Mix the sherry, soy sauce and salt in a jug and pour it all over the fish. Steam vigorously for 15 minutes and serve.

FISH PULAO

1 tablespoon ground coriander
2 teaspoons ground cumin
½ teaspoon ground turmeric
½ teaspoon fenugreek
pinch of ground ginger
2 tablespoons polyunsaturated vegetable oil
750 g/1½–1¾ lb filleted white fish, cut into
    5 cm/2 inch pieces
2 large onions, finely chopped
450 g/1 lb brown rice, washed and soaked for 1
    hour in cold water
2 tablespoons desiccated coconut
2 tablespoons lemon juice

SERVES 4–6
4 servings
Per serving:
Energy 670 kcal/2845 kJ
CHO   90 g (9 units)
Fibre   6 g   **Fat** 17 g   **Protein** 41 g

6 servings
Per serving:
Energy 450 kcal/1895 kJ
CHO   60 g (6 units)
Fibre   5 g   **Fat** 11 g   **Protein** 27 g

Mix the coriander, cumin, turmeric, fenugreek and ginger together. Heat 1 tablespoon of the oil in a large frying pan and fry the spice mixture for about 1 minute. Then place the fish in the pan. Pour in just enough water to cover the fish. Simmer until the fish is cooked, then remove it carefully with a fish slice and keep warm. Reserve the liquid.

Meanwhile, fry the onions in the remaining oil until brown. Drain the rice and add it to the onions. Mix well, then add the reserved fish liquid, the coconut and lemon

juice. Simmer gently until the rice is cooked, adding extra water during cooking when necessary but make sure that when the rice is tender, the liquid has been absorbed.

Place the rice in a warm serving dish. Arrange the fish pieces on top of the rice before serving.

CATALAN COD

25 g/1 oz polyunsaturated margarine
1 onion, sliced
1 garlic clove, crushed
25 g/1 oz wholemeal flour
1 × 400 g (14 oz) can tomatoes
1 tablespoon tomato purée
50 g/2 oz stuffed olives, cut in half
salt
freshly ground black pepper
225 g/8 oz cod steaks

2 tablespoons lemon juice
TO GARNISH
25 g/1 oz hazelnuts, chopped
chopped parsley

SERVES 2
Per serving:
Energy 270 kcal/1125 kJ
CHO 14 g (1.5 units)
Fibre 4 g **Fat** 13 g **Protein** 22 g

Melt the margarine in a saucepan and cook the onion and garlic until soft. Add the flour and continue to cook for 1 minute. Stir in the tomatoes and add the tomato purée. Bring to the boil, stirring constantly, then add the olives and salt and pepper.

Place the cod steaks in a greased shallow ovenproof dish. Sprinkle with the lemon juice and salt and pepper. Pour the tomato sauce over the fish, cover with foil and cook in a preheated moderate oven (180°C, 350°F, Gas Mark 4) for 25 minutes. Serve garnished with hazelnuts and parsley. *Illustrated on page 84.*

OTAK-OTAK

4 small fish (e.g. trout, mackerel, codling), cleaned, heads and back bones removed
¼ teaspoon coriander seeds
salt
freshly ground black pepper
1 egg, beaten
3 tablespoons milk
1 small onion, grated
1 garlic clove, crushed
25 g/1 oz polyunsaturated margarine, melted

cabbage leaves for steaming
TO GARNISH
sliced tomatoes
red peppers, cut into rings

SERVES 4
Per serving:
Energy 420 kcal/1770 kJ
CHO 0 g (0 units)
Fibre 0 g **Fat** 18 g **Protein** 60 g

Wash and dry the fish thoroughly. Then place the fish with the skin side uppermost on a work surface and beat gently with a wooden spoon. This loosens the skin. Turn the fish over and very carefully cut away the raw flesh, leaving the skin intact. Finely chop the fish. Mix the flesh with the coriander, salt, pepper, egg and milk. Add the onion and garlic to the fish with the melted margarine. Spoon the mixture back over the fish skins, then fold to look like the whole fish again.

Wrap each fish in large cabbage leaves and place in a steamer or a large dish over a pan of boiling water. Cover the steamer or dish very tightly and steam for 25–30 minutes until tender. Unwrap and garnish with the tomatoes and red peppers.

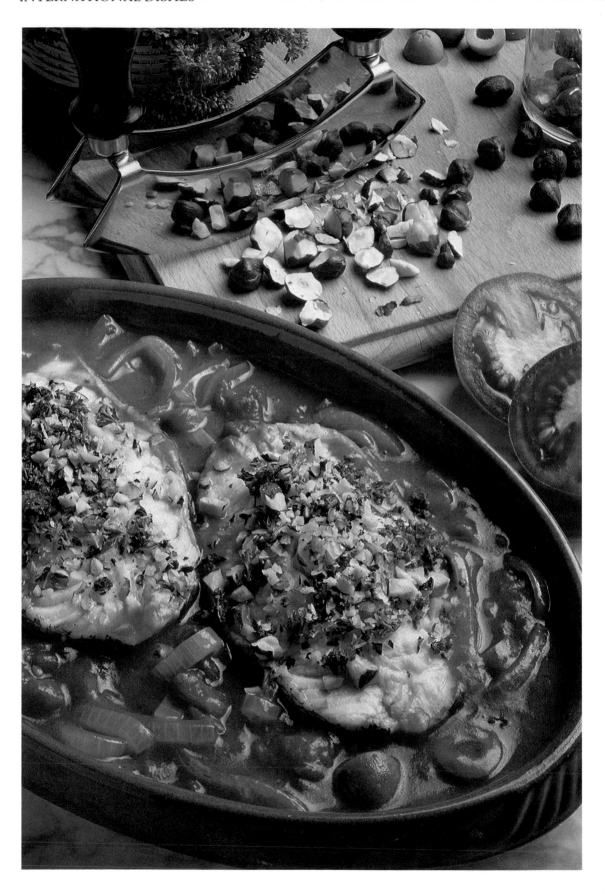

MEDITERRANEAN LIVER

450 g / 1 lb lamb's liver, washed, trimmed and
    thinly sliced
1 onion, finely sliced
1 green pepper, cored, seeded and sliced
1 red pepper, cored, seeded and sliced
1 garlic clove, crushed
1 × 400 g (14 oz) can tomatoes
salt and freshly ground black pepper

TO GARNISH
1 tablespoon chopped parsley

SERVES 4
Per serving:
Energy 220 kcal / 920 kJ
CHO 5 g (0.5 units)
Fibre 1 g   **Fat** 11 g   **Protein** 24 g

Layer the liver in a shallow casserole with the onion, green and red peppers and the garlic. Pour over the canned tomatoes with the juice and season to taste with salt and pepper. Cover and cook in a preheated moderate oven (180°C, 350°F, Gas Mark 4) for 1 hour. Remove, adjust seasoning and sprinkle with the finely chopped parsley.

ITALIAN BAKED BEANS WITH BACON

225 g / 8 oz dried haricot beans, soaked
    overnight in 600 ml / 1 pint water
1 tablespoon polyunsaturated vegetable oil
100 g / 4 oz streaky bacon, rinded and diced
1 onion, chopped
1 garlic clove, crushed
1 tablespoon chopped fresh or 1½ teaspoons
    dried sage

2 tablespoons chopped parsley
1 tablespoon lemon juice
1 tablespoon grated lemon rind
1 bay leaf
salt and freshly ground black pepper
1 tablespoon tomato purée
TO GARNISH
fresh sage or parsley

SERVES 4–6

4 servings
Per serving:
Energy 300 kcal / 1255 kJ
CHO 25 g (2.5 units)
Fibre 14 g   **Fat** 14 g   **Protein** 16 g

6 servings
Per serving:
Energy 200 kcal / 835 kJ
CHO 20 g (2 units)
Fibre 9 g   **Fat** 9 g   **Protein** 10 g

Put the beans and soaking water into a saucepan, bring to the boil and boil for 10 minutes.

Heat the oil in a saucepan and cook the bacon, onion and garlic for 5 minutes or until lightly browned. Add the beans with their liquid and all the remaining ingredients. Bring to the boil. Transfer the mixture to a casserole, cover and bake in a preheated moderate oven (180°C, 350°F, Gas Mark 4) for 2–3 hours or until the beans are tender and most of the liquid has been absorbed.

Alternatively, cook on top of the cooker in a covered saucepan until the beans are tender. Serve hot, garnished with sage or parsley.

CATALAN COD (P. 83)

CÔTES DE PORC AUX LENTILLES

450 g/1 lb green lentils, soaked for 1 hour in
  cold water
1 bay leaf
2 onions
1 whole clove
salt
freshly ground black pepper
6 pork chops, trimmed of fat
4 sage leaves, trimmed
6 small sausages

15 g/½ oz polyunsaturated margarine
2 carrots, scraped and diced
about 600 ml/1 pint chicken stock

SERVES 6
Per serving:
Energy 520 kcal/2200 kJ
CHO 40 g (4 units)
Fibre 14 g **Fat** 18 g **Protein** 47 g

Rinse the lentils under cold running water and pick them over carefully to remove any grit or discoloured lentils. Place in a large pan with the bay leaf and 1 onion stuck with the clove. Cover with water, bring to the boil and simmer for 1 hour. Add salt and pepper to taste halfway through the cooking time.

Meanwhile, sprinkle the chops with the sage and salt and pepper to taste. Grill the chops for 10 minutes until browned on all sides. Prick the sausage skins with a fork and grill.

Melt the margarine in a flameproof casserole. Chop the remaining onion and put in the casserole with the carrots and fry over a brisk heat for 10 minutes until lightly coloured, stirring constantly.

Drain the lentils, then add to the casserole with the chops. Cover with the stock and bring to the boil. Lower the heat, cover and cook gently for 1 hour or until the chops are tender.

Taste and adjust the seasoning. Remove the chops and sausages from the casserole and arrange around the edge of a warmed serving platter. Pile the lentils in the centre. Serve immediately.

FABONADE

25 g/1 oz polyunsaturated margarine
1 onion, finely chopped
150 g/5 oz ham, diced
4 garlic cloves, crushed
1 kg/2 lb broad beans, shelled
2–3 sprigs savory
150 ml/¼ pint water
salt and freshly ground black pepper
3 egg yolks

2 tablespoons vinegar or lemon juice
TO GARNISH
chopped parsley

SERVES 6
Per serving:
Energy 270 kcal/1150 kJ
CHO 20 g (2 units)
Fibre 9 g **Fat** 13 g **Protein** 22 g

Melt the margarine in a heavy pan, add the onion and ham and cook gently for a few minutes. Add the garlic, beans and savory, then the water, and salt and pepper to taste. Mix well. Bring to the boil, then lower the heat, cover and simmer for 20–30 minutes until the beans are tender.

Discard the savory. Mix the egg yolks and vinegar or lemon juice together, then stir slowly into the beans. Heat through, but do not allow to boil. Taste and adjust the seasoning, then transfer to a warmed serving dish and garnish with parsley. Serve immediately.

VITELLO TONNATO

1 × 50 g (2 oz) can anchovy fillets, drained
1.75 kg/4 lb fillet of veal joint, trimmed and
  gristle removed
4–5 cloves (optional)
1 medium onion
2 carrots, scraped and sliced
1 celery stick, chopped
salt

freshly ground black pepper
SAUCE
1 × 200 g (7 oz) can tuna fish, drained and
  flaked
juice of 1 lemon
1–2 tablespoons capers
TO GARNISH
1 lemon, sliced

SERVES 6–8
6 servings
Per serving:
Energy 340 kcal/1440 kJ
CHO 0 g (0 units)
Fibre 0 g   **Fat** 14 g   **Protein** 52 g

8 servings
Per serving:
Energy 295 kcal/1235 kJ
CHO 0 g (0 units)
Fibre 0 g   **Fat** 12 g   **Protein** 44 g

The sauce is often made ahead and allowed to stand for 24 hours, so the flavours blend more readily. Do not throw away the cooking liquid and vegetables. Add extra vegetables, rice or pasta and serve as a soup at a separate meal.

Use half the anchovies to cover the veal. Press the cloves, if used, into the onion.

Put the veal into a large saucepan, add the vegetables and just enough water to cover the meat. Add a little salt and pepper but remember that anchovies are very salty. Cover the saucepan and simmer very gently for 1½ hours.

While the meat is cooking, prepare the sauce. Chop the remaining anchovies. Mix the tuna with the anchovies; pound or blend to a smooth mixture. Add the lemon juice as desired. Lastly add the capers.

Remove the meat from the liquid, carve into thin slices, top with the sauce. Arrange the lemon slices over the sauce. Serve with boiled potatoes and a green salad.

MEXICAN CHICKEN

1 tablespoon polyunsaturated vegetable oil
1.5 kg/3 lb boiling chicken, cut into 8 pieces
2 onions, chopped
3 garlic cloves, chopped
2 teaspoons chilli powder, or to taste
600 ml/1 pint chicken stock
1 × 225 g (8 oz) can tomatoes
salt
freshly ground black pepper

1 × 450 g (1 lb) can red kidney beans, rinsed
  and drained

SERVES 4
Per serving:
Energy 420 kcal/1765 kJ
CHO 20 g (2 units)
Fibre 9 g   **Fat** 11 g   **Protein** 63 g

Heat the oil in a flameproof casserole. Add the chicken pieces, onions and garlic and fry until lightly browned. Add the chilli powder gradually and fry gently for a further 2 minutes. Pour in the stock and then the tomatoes with their juice. Bring to the boil and skim. Add salt and pepper to taste. Simmer gently for about 2 hours or until tender.

About 10 minutes before the chicken is ready, add the beans. Stir well and adjust the seasoning. (Alternatively, the beans may be heated and served separately.)

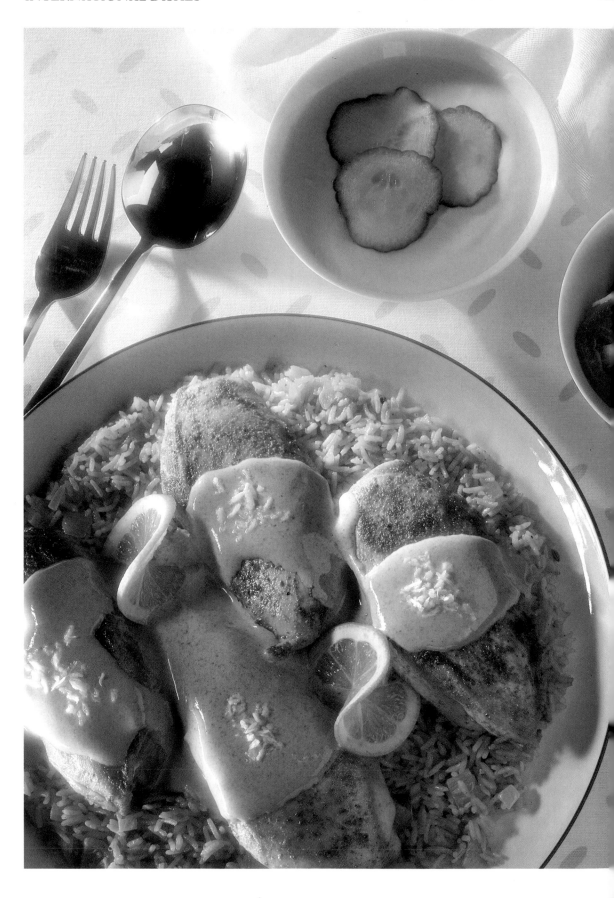

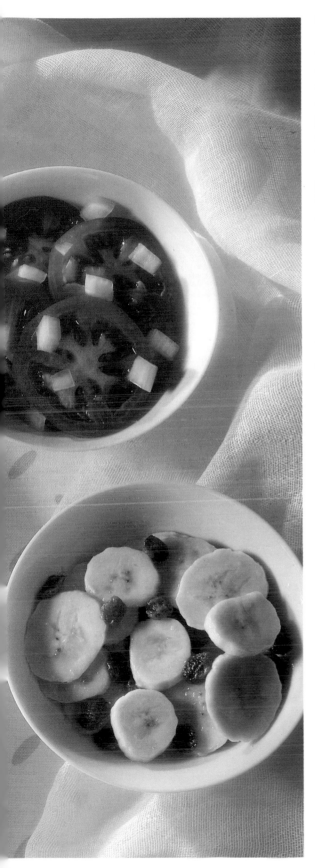

SPICED CHICKEN

½ teaspoon ground coriander
½ teaspoon chilli powder
½ teaspoon garam masala
pinch of salt
2 tablespoons lemon juice
4 boneless chicken breasts, about 100 g/4 oz
  each, skinned
polyunsaturated vegetable oil
SAUCE
300 ml/½ pint plain unsweetened yogurt
½ teaspoon ground ginger
1 teaspoon curry powder
1 tablespoon cayenne pepper
1 garlic clove, crushed
1 bay leaf
1 tablespoon tomato purée
1 tablespoon grated lemon rind
TO GARNISH
parsley sprigs
lemon slices

SERVES 4
Per serving:
Energy 180 kcal/755 kJ
CHO 5 g (0.5 units)
Fibre 0 g **Fat** 6 g **Protein** 25 g

Combine the coriander, chilli powder, garam masala, salt and lemon juice. Prick the chicken breasts all over with a fork and rub in the spice and lemon mixture. Leave to marinate for 4–5 hours.

Drain the chicken breasts and fry them in oil over a moderate heat until they are brown all over and cooked through. Transfer to a serving dish and keep warm.

Meanwhile mix together all the ingredients for the sauce and warm over a gentle heat, stirring constantly. Remove the bay leaf and pour the sauce over the fried chicken breasts.

Garnish with parsley and lemon slices. Serve with pilau rice, grated coconut, sultanas and a selection of other accompaniments to taste.

DOLMAS

350 g / 12 oz minced beef
1 onion, finely chopped
50 g / 2 oz mushrooms, peeled and sliced
1 tomato, skinned and chopped
1 teaspoon oregano
1 tablespoon tomato purée
salt
freshly ground black pepper
8 cabbage leaves, washed and trimmed
250 ml / 8 fl oz tomato juice

1 teaspoon cornflour
1 tablespoon finely chopped mint
TO GARNISH
tomato slices

SERVES 4
Per serving:
Energy 220 kcal / 915 kJ
CHO 5 g (0.5 units)
Fibre 1 g **Fat** 14 g **Protein** 17 g

In a non-stick frying pan cook the minced beef, onion and mushrooms until brown – about 4 minutes. Stir in the tomato, oregano and tomato purée; season to taste with salt and pepper.

Blanch the cabbage leaves in boiling salted water for 3–4 minutes and drain.

Divide the meat mixture between the cabbage leaves and roll up (secure with cocktail sticks if wished).

Blend together the tomato juice and cornflour. Place in a small saucepan and bring to the boil, stirring. Add the chopped mint. Pour half the sauce into an ovenproof dish. Arrange the stuffed cabbage leaves on top. Cover tightly. Bake in a preheated moderate oven (180°C, 350°F, Gas Mark 4) for 1 hour.

Warm the remaining sauce through and pour over the cabbage leaves. Garnish with the tomato slices. *Illustrated on pages 56–7.*

MEXICAN HAMBURGERS

450 g / 1 lb minced beef
1 onion, finely grated (optional)
1 egg, lightly beaten
salt
freshly ground black pepper
2 teaspoons Worcestershire sauce
SAUCE
2 teaspoons polyunsaturated vegetable oil
2 medium onions, minced
2 garlic cloves, minced
2 small green peppers, cored, seeded and sliced
  in rings

50 g / 2 oz mushrooms, chopped
1 × 400 g (14 oz) can tomatoes
2 teaspoons dried marjoram or oregano
dash of hot chilli sauce

SERVES 4
Per serving:
Energy 275 kcal / 1055 kJ
CHO 12 g (1 unit)
Fibre 2 g **Fat** 14 g **Protein** 24 g

Mix the beef with the onion, if used. Mix in the egg, salt and pepper to taste and the Worcestershire sauce. Divide into four equal pieces and shape into hamburgers about 2 cm / ¾ inch thick.

To make the sauce, heat the oil in a frying pan. Add the onions and garlic and fry until they are golden. Add the pepper rings and continue cooking for 15 minutes. Stir in the mushrooms, tomatoes with their can juice and the marjoram or oregano. Season to taste with the chilli sauce, salt and pepper. Cover and continue cooking for a further 10 minutes.

Meanwhile place the hamburgers on the rack of a grill pan. Cook under a preheated hot grill until rare or medium, to your taste. Arrange the hamburgers on a hot serving dish and pour the sauce over them. Serve with a crisp green salad.

CHICKEN DOPIAZZA

3 onions, thinly sliced
2 tablespoons polyunsaturated vegetable oil
1/4 teaspoon garlic powder
1 tablespoon coriander seeds
1 tablespoon ground cumin
1/2 teaspoon ground turmeric
1 teaspoon ground ginger
1/2–1 teaspoon chilli powder
350 g/12 oz fresh tomatoes, halved
350 g/12 oz small new potatoes, washed

freshly ground black pepper
750 g/1 1/2–1 3/4 lb chicken meat, cut into
    2.5 cm/1 inch cubes
salt

SERVES 4
Per serving:
Energy 375 kcal/1620 kJ
CHO 19 g (2 units)
Fibre 3 g **Fat** 12 g **Protein** 40 g

Fry the onions in the oil in a large pan until they are golden brown. Mix the garlic powder with the spices and a little pepper. Add the spice mixture to the pan with the chicken meat. Fry, stirring all the time, for about 1 minute.

Pour in sufficient water to cover the chicken and add salt to taste. Bring to the boil, cover and simmer for 45 minutes or until the chicken is nearly cooked. Add water during cooking, if necessary, to ensure the mixture does not become dry. Then add the tomatoes and potatoes and continue to simmer until the vegetables are cooked.

PORK CHOP SUEY

2 tablespoons soy sauce
1 tablespoon dry sherry
2 teaspoons cornflour
225 g/8 oz pork fillet (or chicken meat), cut
    into 2.5 cm/1 inch slices
100 g/4 oz fresh bean-sprouts, rinsed and
    thoroughly dried
1 tablespoon polyunsaturated vegetable oil
2 spring onions, cut into 2.5 cm/1 inch lengths
1 slice ginger root, peeled and finely chopped
1 small green pepper, cored, seeded and cut into
    1 cm/1/2 inch pieces
2–3 tomatoes, cut into 1 cm/1/2 inch pieces

a few cauliflower or broccoli florets, cut into
    1 cm/1/2 inch pieces
1–2 carrots, cut into 1 cm/1/2 inch pieces
50 g/2 oz French beans, cut into 1 cm/1/2 inch
    pieces
1 teaspoon salt
stock or water, if necessary

SERVES 4
Per serving:
Energy 155 kcal/640 kJ
CHO 6 g (0.5 units)
Fibre 1 g **Fat** 7 g **Protein** 13 g

Mix together the soy sauce, sherry and cornflour, and stir in the meat until each slice is coated with the mixture.

Heat about half the oil in a wok or frying pan and stir-fry the meat slices for about 1 minute, stirring constantly, then remove with a perforated spoon and put them on one side.

Heat the remaining oil, add the spring onions and ginger root, followed by the remaining vegetables and the salt. Stir for about 1 minute and add the meat. Blend everything well and moisten with a little stock or water if necessary. Serve with boiled rice.

SINGAPORE SPARE-RIBS

1 medium onion, chopped
1 garlic clove, chopped
3 tablespoons wine vinegar
1 tablespoon soy sauce
1 teaspoon sesame oil
¼ teaspoon aniseed
450 ml/¾ pint water
1.5 kg/3 lb pork spare-ribs
1 medium mango, peeled and diced

1 small pineapple, peeled, cored and cut into
 2.5 cm/1 inch fingers

SERVES 4
Per serving:
Energy 500 kcal/2080 kJ
CHO 10 g (1 unit)
Fibre 2 g   **Fat** 40 g   **Protein** 22 g

Combine the onion, garlic, vinegar, soy sauce, oil, spice and water in a large pan, then add the spare-ribs. Bring to the boil, lower the heat, cover and simmer for 1 hour or until the spare-ribs are tender, turning them after 30 minutes.

Remove the pork from the pan and cut into separate ribs. Boil the liquid in the pan until reduced to one-third of its original volume. Taste for seasoning. Add the fruit and simmer for 2–3 minutes, then pour over the ribs.

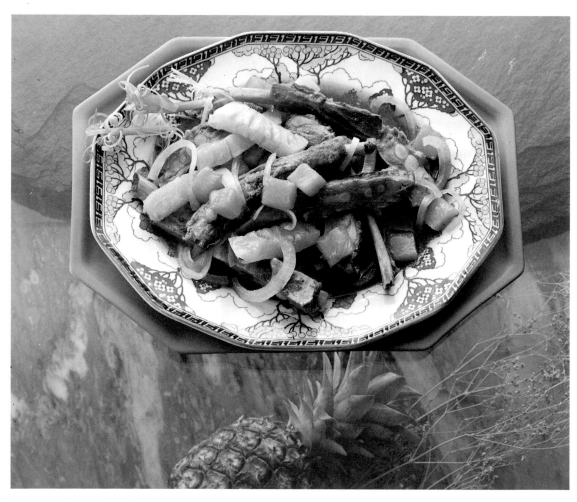

ABOVE: SINGAPORE SPARE–RIBS

OPPOSITE: LEEKS WITH ORANGE AND THYME (P. 23); BELOW: COURGETTES NIÇOISES (P. 94)

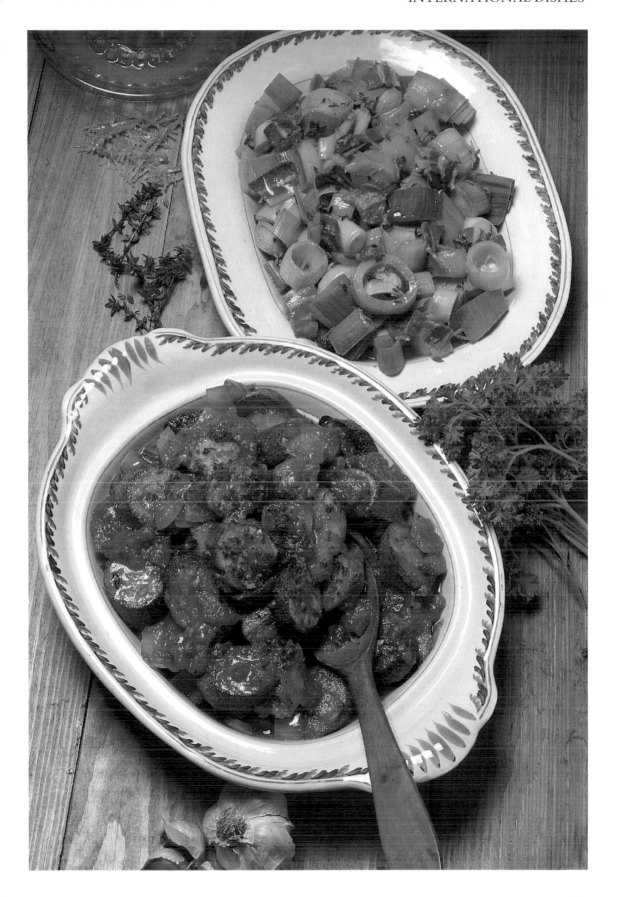

COURGETTES NIÇOISES

2 tablespoons low-fat spread
1 onion, chopped
1 garlic clove, crushed (optional)
450 g/1 lb courgettes, sliced
225 g/8 oz tomatoes, sliced
salt
freshly ground black pepper

TO GARNISH
1 tablespoon chopped parsley

SERVES 4
Per serving:
Energy 60 kcal/245 kJ
CHO 7 g (1 unit)
Fibre 3 g **Fat** 3 g **Protein** 1 g

Melt the spread in a frying pan, and fry the onion, garlic (if used) and courgettes for 5 minutes or until lightly browned, turning occasionally. Stir in the tomatoes, salt and pepper.

Cover the pan and cook gently for 5–10 minutes, stirring occasionally, or until the tomatoes are reduced to a pulp and the courgettes are just tender.

Turn into a serving dish and garnish with parsley. *Illustrated on page 93.*

MEDITERRANEAN LENTIL STEW

2 tablespoons polyunsaturated vegetable oil
2 onions, chopped
2 gloves garlic, crushed
2 celery sticks, sliced
4 small courgettes, sliced
4 tomatoes, quartered
900 ml/1½ pints water or stock
¼ teaspoon ground coriander
salt
freshly ground black pepper

225 g/8 oz brown lentils, soaked for 1 hour in cold water
TO GARNISH
2 tablespoons chopped parsley (optional)

SERVES 4
Per serving:
Energy 260 kcal/1100 kJ
CHO 35 g (3.5 units)
Fibre 8 g **Fat** 8 g **Protein** 14 g

Heat the oil in a large pan. Add the onions, garlic, celery and courgettes and fry gently for 10 minutes until lightly browned, stirring frequently.

Add the tomatoes, water or stock, coriander, salt and pepper to taste. Bring to the boil. Add the lentils, then cover and simmer the pot for 1–1½ hours or until the lentils are tender.

Alternatively, transfer the ingredients to a casserole, cover and bake in a preheated moderate oven (180°C, 350°F, Gas Mark 4) for 1½–2 hours.

Sprinkle with the chopped parsley, if liked, and serve hot.

HORENSO TAMAGO MAKI

350 g/12 oz spinach
1 teaspoon soy sauce
2 eggs, beaten
pinch of salt
polyunsaturated vegetable oil

SERVES 4
Per serving:
Energy 90 kcal/380 kJ
CHO 5 g (0.5 units)
Fibre 0 g **Fat** 6 g **Protein** 6 g

Drop the spinach into boiling water and simmer for about 1½ minutes or until the leaves collapse and turn bright green. Drain and rinse twice under cold water, then press the spinach to extract the excess water. Trim off any hard stalks. Sprinkle the spinach with the soy sauce. Divide into two portions and shape each into a long roll.

Mix the eggs with the salt. Add a little oil to a 20 cm/8 inch frying pan and heat.

Pour in half the egg mixture and tilt the pan so that the bottom is evenly coated. Cook until the egg mixture is set. Turn out on to a cloth.

Place one of the spinach rolls at the edge of the omelette and roll up firmly to enclose the spinach. Repeat with the remaining egg mixture and spinach roll. Cool slightly, then cut across the rolled omelettes into 2.5 cm/1 inch slices. Serve cold, with light soy sauce as a dip. See p. 97.

SPICY CHICK PEAS

300 g/11 oz dried chick peas, soaked overnight
   in cold water
salt and freshly ground black pepper
6 rashers streaky bacon, rinded and diced
2 onions, chopped
1 garlic clove, crushed
1 red pepper, cored, seeded and chopped
1 small dried red chilli, crumbled

½ teaspoon dried oregano
150 ml/¼ pint canned tomato sauce

SERVES 4
Per serving:

Energy	380 kcal/1600 kJ		
CHO	40 g (4 units)		
Fibre	11 g	**Fat** 16 g	**Protein** 20 g

Drain the chick peas and place in a pan with a little salt. Pour over enough water just to cover. Bring to the boil, boil for 10 minutes and simmer, uncovered, for about 45 minutes until the chick peas are cooked and tender. Drain.

Place the bacon in a pan and fry until the fat runs. Add the onions, garlic and red pepper and fry until soft. Stir in the chilli, oregano, tomato sauce and chick peas. Add the pepper to taste. Simmer for 10 minutes, stirring occasionally.

SPICED FRUIT AND VEGETABLES

1 onion, chopped
4 celery sticks
1 tablespoon vegetable oil
1 tablespoon curry powder
1 tablespoon plain flour
300 ml/½ pint light stock or water
1 × 2.5 cm/1 inch piece fresh root ginger
2 tablespoons lemon juice
2 tablespoons grated lemon rind
1 × 400 g (14 oz) can unsweetened apricot
   halves, drained

2 bananas, peeled and thickly sliced
450 g/1 lb cooking apples, peeled, cored and
   quartered
100 g/4 oz raisins
150 ml/¼ pint plain unsweetened yogurt

SERVES 6
Per serving:

Energy	145 kcal/605 kJ		
CHO	28 g (3 units)		
Fibre	5 g	**Fat** 3 g	**Protein** 3 g

Fry the onion and celery in the oil until golden. Stir in the curry powder and flour and cook gently for 2–3 minutes, stirring constantly. Mix the stock or water with the ginger and gradually stir into the pan. Add the lemon juice, rind, apricots, bananas, apples and raisins. Stir well and cook, covered, over a low heat until the fruit is tender. Just before serving, stir in the yogurt.

TAGLIATELLE WITH TUNA

350 g/12 oz wholemeal tagliatelle
1 × 200 g/7 oz can tuna fish
1 medium onion, chopped
100 g/4 oz mushrooms, sliced
salt and freshly ground black pepper
2 tablespoons tomato purée

SERVES 4
Per serving:
Energy 440 kcal/1870 kJ
CHO 65 g (6.5 units)
Fibre 4 g   **Fat** 11 g   **Protein** 22 g

Cook the tagliatelle in a large pan of boiling water until tender.

Meanwhile, drain the oil from the tuna fish into a saucepan. Cook the onion in the oil until tender, then add the mushrooms and cook until soft. Season to taste.

When the tagliatelle is cooked, drain well and return to the pan. Flake the tuna and add with the onion and mushrooms. Add the tomato purée and mix all the ingredients together over a low heat. Adjust the seasoning and serve immediately.

WHOLEMEAL VEGETABLE SAMOSAS

3 carrots, scraped and diced
4 medium potatoes, peeled and diced
½ teaspoon salt
½ teaspoon ground cumin
½ teaspoon ground coriander
½ teaspoon ground turmeric
½ teaspoon chilli powder
about 120 ml/4 fl oz boiling water
5–6 spinach leaves, finely chopped
PASTRY
350 g/12 oz self-raising wholemeal flour

½ teaspoon salt
75 g/3 oz polyunsaturated margarine
about 200 ml/⅓ pint cold water
a little milk

SERVES 4
Per serving:
Energy 480 kcal/2020 kJ
CHO 72 g (7 units)
Fibre 11 g   **Fat** 17 g   **Protein** 13 g

Put the carrots and potatoes into a saucepan with the salt, spices and boiling water. Cover tightly and simmer for 10 minutes. Shake the pan occasionally to prevent the vegetables sticking. Add the spinach leaves and simmer for a further 5 minutes, adding a little more boiling water if necessary.

Meanwhile, make the pastry. Sift the flour and salt into a large mixing bowl, tipping in any bran left in the sieve. Rub in the margarine until the mixture resembles fine crumbs. Stir in enough water to make a soft dough, then shape the dough into a ball and divide into three portions.

Put one-third of the dough on to a floured board and roll out into a rectangle about 18 × 23 cm/7 × 9 inch. Spread one-third of the vegetable mixture along the length of the rectangle. Bring the long edges together, moistening each edge with a little milk to make them stick. Dust with a little flour and cut into the rectangle to make three squares. Repeat with the remaining dough and vegetable mixture. Place the samosas on a greased and floured baking sheet. Cook in a preheated moderately hot oven (200°C, 400°F, Gas Mark 6) for 25 minutes.

Serve hot with an accompanying salad.

CENTRE: NASU NO KARASHI; HORENSO TAMAGO MAKI (p. 94–5)

NASU NO KARASHI

1 medium aubergine, cut crossways into 5 mm/
   ¼ inch thick slices
750 ml/1¼ pints water
1 tablespoon salt
DRESSING
1 teaspoon dry mustard
3 tablespoons light soy sauce

1 tablespoon wine vinegar
1 drop artificial sweetener

SERVES 4
Per serving:
Energy	20 kcal/85 kJ
CHO	0 g (0 units)

Fibre 1 g   **Fat** 0 g   **Protein** 1 g

Cut the aubergine slices into quarters. Soak in the water, with the salt, for 1 hour.

Meanwhile mix together all the dressing ingredients.

Drain the aubergine and pat dry with paper towels. Arrange in a glass serving dish and pour over the dressing. Cover and chill for several hours or overnight.

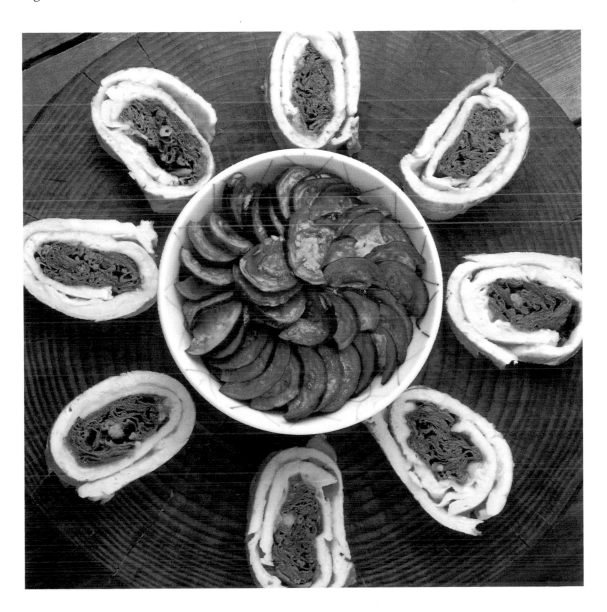

Children's Recipes

BACON-TOPPED LIVER

350 g/12 oz lamb's or pig's liver, cut into 8
   thick slices
salt and freshly ground black pepper
1 × 425 g (15 oz) can tomatoes
6 tablespoons wholemeal breadcrumbs mixed
   with dried parsley and dried thyme
2 tablespoons water
6 rashers bacon, rinded and halved
15 g/½ oz polyunsaturated margarine

TO GARNISH
chopped parsley

SERVES 4
Per serving:
Energy 350 kcal/1480 kJ
CHO   10 g (1 unit)
Fibre   2 g   **Fat** 23 g   **Protein** 24 g

Put half the liver in a casserole or oven-proof dish and season well with salt and pepper. Cover with the tomatoes, reserving a little of the juice, then sprinkle with half of the breadcrumb mixture. Cover with the remaining liver, pour over the reserved tomato juice and the water. Add salt and pepper to taste. Lay the pieces of bacon on top. Sprinkle with the remaining breadcrumb mixture, dot with the margarine and cover the casserole. Cook in a preheated moderately hot oven (190°C, 375°F, Gas Mark 5) for 30 minutes. Remove the lid and return to the oven for a further 20–30 minutes or until the liver is tender. Garnish with parsley.

FISH STEAKS WITH ORANGE SAUCE

1 kg/2 lb cod or haddock, cut into 4 steaks
900 ml/1½ pints cold fish stock
15 g/½ oz polyunsaturated margarine
1 teaspoon polyunsaturated vegetable oil
1 small onion, finely chopped
175 ml/6 fl oz frozen concentrated orange juice
2 teaspoons chopped tarragon
2 teaspoons chopped parsley
salt
freshly ground black pepper

2 teaspoons cornflour
1 tablespoon water
TO GARNISH
8 orange segments, pith removed

SERVES 4
Per serving:
Energy 250 kcal/1050 kJ
CHO   5 g (0.5 units)
Fibre   0 g   **Fat** 9 g   **Protein** 35 g

Rinse the fish under cold running water and dry it with absorbent kitchen paper. Trim off any fins, then place in a lightly buttered flameproof dish. Poor over the fish stock, bring to the boil, reduce the heat immediately and poach for 10 minutes. Remove the fish from the liquid on to a warm serving dish, remove the skin and bones and keep hot. Strain off 150 ml/¼ pint of the liquid and reserve.

Heat the margarine and oil in a saucepan and cook the onion gently. Stir in the orange juice, reserved fish liquid, herbs and salt and pepper to taste. Bring to the boil and simmer for 3 minutes. Mix the cornflour with the water, stir into the sauce and bring slowly to the boil, stirring constantly. Remove from the heat. Taste and adjust the seasoning, then pour the sauce over the fish steaks. Garnish with orange segments.

MACARONI CRUNCH

1 tablespoon polyunsaturated vegetable oil
2 onions, chopped
225 g/8 oz wholemeal macaroni
1 × 400 g (14 oz) can tomatoes
225 g/8 oz Cheddar cheese, grated
2 tablespoons Bran Flakes

SERVES 4
Per serving:
Energy 480 kcal/2000 kJ
CHO 45 g (4.5 units)
Fibre 1 g **Fat** 23 g **Protein** 22 g

Heat the oil in a frying pan and fry the onions for 10 minutes. In a deep casserole dish, arrange layers of onion, uncooked macaroni and tomatoes, together with all but 2 tablespoons of the cheese. Mix the Bran Flakes with remaining cheese for the topping and bake in a preheated moderate oven (160°C, 325°F, Gas Mark 3) for 1 hour.

CHEESE AND WALNUT BURGERS

175 g/6 oz shelled walnuts
50 g/2 oz wholemeal bread, roughly cubed
50 g/2 oz low-fat cheese, grated
1 onion, grated
salt
freshly ground black pepper
1 egg
1 tablespoon tomato purée
polyunsaturated vegetable oil for shallow frying

TO GARNISH
tomato slices
watercress

SERVES 4
Per serving:
Energy 315 kcal/1315 kJ
CHO 8 g (1 unit)
Fibre 4 g **Fat** 26 g **Protein** 11 g

Reserve 50 g/2 oz of the walnuts for the coating and put the remainder into a blender. Add the bread cubes and grind coarsely. Transfer to a bowl, add the cheese, onion and salt and pepper to taste and stir well. Beat the egg with the tomato purée. Add to the nut mixture and combine well.

Divide the mixture into four on a lightly floured surface. Shape into burgers, about 9 cm/3½ inch in diameter and 1 cm/½ inch thick. Chop the reserved walnuts and press into both sides of the burgers.

Heat a little oil in a frying pan, add the burgers and fry for about 5 minutes until browned on both sides, turning once. Alternatively, place the burgers on a lightly greased baking sheet and bake in a preheated moderately hot oven (200°C, 400°F, Gas Mark 6) for 20 minutes or until browned.

Serve hot or cold, garnished with tomato slices and watercress.

SMOKED COD JUMBLE

225 g/8 oz wholemeal macaroni
25 g/1 oz polyunsaturated margarine
3 tablespoons milk
350 g/12 oz smoked cod or haddock fillets,
    skinned and cut into 2.5 cm/1 inch cubes
4 tomatoes, chopped
6 spring onions, trimmed and chopped
salt and freshly ground black pepper

SERVES 4
Per serving:
Energy 350 kcal/1515 kJ
CHO 50 g (5 units)
Fibre 3 g   **Fat** 6 g   **Protein** 25 g

Cook the macaroni for 10–15 minutes in plenty of boiling slightly salted water. Drain well.

Melt the margarine in a saucepan. Add the milk and fish, cover and cook very gently for 10 minutes, or until the fish is tender. Remove the lid, add the cooked macaroni, tomatoes and spring onions. Season with salt and pepper. Stir the mixture lightly to avoid breaking up the fish, and reheat well.

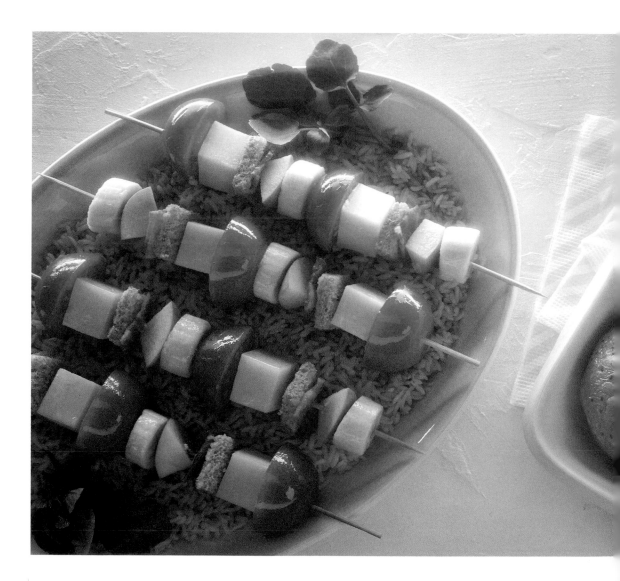

BACON-STUFFED POTATOES

4 large potatoes, well scrubbed
25 g/1 oz polyunsaturated margarine
75 g/3 oz bacon, rinded, chopped and grilled
2 tablespoons skimmed milk
25 g/1 oz walnuts, chopped
50 g/2 oz Cheddar cheese, grated
1 tablespoon chopped parsley
salt and freshly ground black pepper

SERVES 4
Per serving:
Energy 290 kcal/1225 kJ
CHO 25 g (2.5 units)
Fibre 3 g **Fat** 16 g **Protein** 12 g

Prick the potatoes with a fork and bake in a preheated moderately hot oven (200°C, 400°F, Gas Mark 6) for 1–1½ hours.

When cooked, cut off the tops of the potatoes lengthwise and scoop out the centres, taking care to keep the skins intact.

Mash the potato in a bowl, and add the margarine, bacon, milk, nuts, cheese, parsley, salt and pepper. Fill the potato shells with the mixture and bake in a preheated moderately hot oven (190°C, 375°F, Gas Mark 5) for 15 minutes.

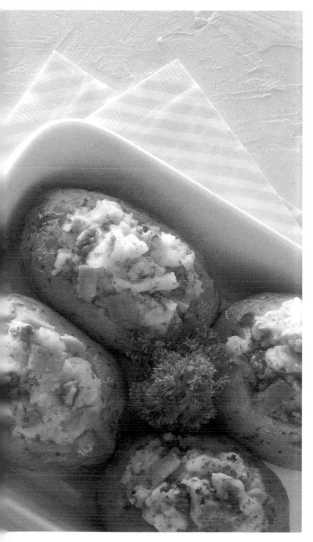

FRUIT AND CHEESE KEBABS

225 g/8 oz Cheddar cheese, cubed
4 tomatoes, cut into quarters
4 slices wholemeal bread, spread with
    polyunsaturated margarine and cut into
    squares
2 rashers streaky bacon, rinded and cut into
    quarters
1 banana, peeled and sliced
1 dessert apple, unpeeled, cored and cubed
polyunsaturated margarine, melted

SERVES 4
Per serving:
Energy 370 kcal/1530 kJ
CHO 15 g (1.5 units)
Fibre 4 g **Fat** 25 g **Protein** 18 g

Place cubes of cheese, quarters of tomato, squares of wholemeal bread, bacon and fruit alternately on to skewers. Brush the kebabs all over with the melted margarine and cook under a preheated hot grill for approximately 3 minutes, turning once. Serve with brown rice.

LEFT: FRUIT AND CHEESE KEBABS; RIGHT:
BACON-STUFFED POTATOES

NOODLES WITH COTTAGE CHEESE

150 g / 6 oz wholemeal noodles
salt and freshly ground black pepper
150 g / 5 oz cottage cheese
25 g / 1 oz grated Parmesan cheese
25 g / 1 oz polyunsaturated margarine
2 tablespoons chopped parsley
1 small onion, chopped
2 eggs, beaten

SERVES 4
Per serving:
Energy 300 kcal / 1270 kJ
CHO 30 g (3 units)
Fibre 3 g   **Fat** 14 g   **Protein** 15 g

Cook the noodles in boiling slightly salted water until soft (approximately 20 minutes). Strain and add the remaining ingredients, mixing well. Place the mixture in a lightly greased casserole and bake in a preheated moderate oven (190°C, 375°F, Gas Mark 5) for 20 minutes.

SPAGHETTI WITH TOMATO AND RED PEPPER SAUCE

1 tablespoon polyunsaturated vegetable oil
1 garlic clove, crushed
1 onion, sliced
450 g / 1 lb minced beef
1 × 400 g (14 oz) can tomatoes
1 red pepper, cored, seeded and sliced
1 tablespoon chopped parsley
salt and freshly ground black pepper
350 g / 12 oz wholemeal spaghetti

SERVES 4
Per serving:
Energy 430 kcal / 1795 kJ
CHO 50 g (5 units)
Fibre 4 g   **Fat** 14 g   **Protein** 22 g

Heat the oil in a saucepan and brown the garlic, onion and beef. Add the tomatoes, red pepper and parsley. Cook 5 minutes, then add sufficient hot water to make a sauce. Season with salt and pepper. Simmer the sauce until thickened slightly, stirring occasionally.

Cook the spaghetti for 10–15 minutes in plenty of boiling water, drain and add the sauce.

SAUSAGE HOTPOT

450 g / 1 lb chipolata sausages
1 large onion, chopped
450 g / 1 lb tomatoes, skinned and chopped
2 carrots, peeled and chopped
600 ml / 1 pint beef stock
50 g / 2 oz sweetcorn kernels

SERVES 4
Per serving:
Energy 350 kcal / 1480 kJ
CHO 25 g (2.5 units)
Fibre 5.5 g   **Fat** 19 g   **Protein** 16 g

Cook the sausages under a preheated hot grill for 10 minutes so that fat is drained off. Place in a casserole together with the remaining ingredients. Cover and cook in a moderately hot oven (190°C, 375°F, Gas Mark 5) for 40 minutes.

POTATO AND TOMATO PIE

25 g / 1 oz polyunsaturated margarine
25 g / 1 oz wholemeal flour
300 ml / ½ pint skimmed milk
100 g / 4 oz Cheddar cheese, grated
450 g / 1 lb potatoes, peeled, boiled and thinly sliced
2 onions, sliced
450 g / 1 lb tomatoes, skinned and sliced

salt and freshly ground black pepper
pinch of dried basil

SERVES 4
Per serving:
Energy 325 kcal / 1370 kJ
CHO 35 g (3.5 units)
Fibre 3 g **Fat** 16 g **Protein** 12 g

Melt the margarine in a saucepan, stir in the flour and gradually add the milk. Bring to the boil, stirring continuously, and cook the sauce for 2–3 minutes. Add 50 g / 2 oz of the cheese and stir until melted.

Grease a shallow, ovenproof dish and arrange the potatoes in layers with the onions, tomatoes and cheese sauce, seasoning with salt, pepper and basil between each layer. Finish with a layer of potato, sprinkle with the remaining cheese and bake in a preheated moderate oven (180°C, 350°F, Gas Mark 4) for 45 minutes.

PITTA PARCEL

½ wholemeal pitta bread
50 g / 2 oz tuna fish, drained and flaked
25 g / 1 oz sweetcorn
1 tablespoon tomato purée
2–3 slices cucumber, chopped into small pieces

SERVES 1
Per serving:
Energy 265 kcal / 1110 kJ
CHO 25 g (2.5 units)
Fibre 4 g **Fat** 11 g **Protein** 16 g

Slice a wholemeal pitta in half across the width, and open with a sharp knife to form a pocket. This can be done more easily if the pitta is slightly warmed first. Mix together the tuna, sweetcorn, tomato purée and cucumber and spoon into the pitta. Serve.

QUICK PIZZA GRILL

1 wholemeal roll
polyunsaturated margarine
25 g / 1 oz lean ham, chopped
1 tomato, sliced
1 tablespoon chopped onion (optional)
25 g / 1 oz Cheddar cheese, sliced

SERVES 1
Per serving:
Energy 300 kcal / 1250 kJ
CHO 20 g (2 units)
Fibre 3 g **Fat** 16 g **Protein** 15 g

Split the wholemeal roll in two and spread each half with a little margarine. Divide the ham, tomato and onion (if using) between the two halves, and cover each half with slices of cheese. Cook under a fairly hot grill for 5–10 minutes, or until the cheese has melted and become lightly browned. Serve immediately.

CHOCOLATE CAKE WITH ALMOND SPREAD

100 g/4 oz plain white flour
75 g/3 oz wholemeal flour
175 ml/6 fl oz skimmed milk
65 g/2½ oz dates, chopped
65 g/2½ oz polyunsaturated margarine
1 teaspoon dried yeast
25 g/1 oz cocoa
2 eggs, separated
SPREAD
75 g/3 oz ground almonds
2 tablespoons polyunsaturated vegetable oil
15 g/½ oz dates, chopped
2 tablespoons orange juice
2 teaspoons water

MAKES 1 × 23 cm (9 inch) cake
Total recipe:
Energy 2415 kcal/10145 kJ
CHO 180 g (18 units)
Fibre 12 g **Fat** 165 g **Protein** 58 g

Sieve the flours together into a bowl. Place the milk, dates and margarine in a saucepan and heat until tepid. Remove from the heat and dissolve the yeast in the mixture. Leave for 10 minutes. Stir the cocoa and egg yolks into the yeast mixture, then stir the whole mixture into the flour. Cover the bowl and leave to rise for 30 minutes.

Stir the mixture well and add the stiffly beaten egg whites, folding them in gently until the mixture reaches a soft dropping consistency. Fill the mixture into a 23 cm (9 inch) cake tin lined with non-stick silicone paper, cover and leave to rise for a further 30 minutes. Bake in a preheated moderately hot oven (190°C, 375°F, Gas Mark 5) for 40 minutes. Cool on a wire tray.

To make the spread, mix the almonds and the oil together. Gradually blend the dates with the almonds, orange juice and water. Spread over the cake.

LEFT: TARZAN TREAT (P. 106); RIGHT: CHOCOLATE CAKE WITH ALMOND SPREAD

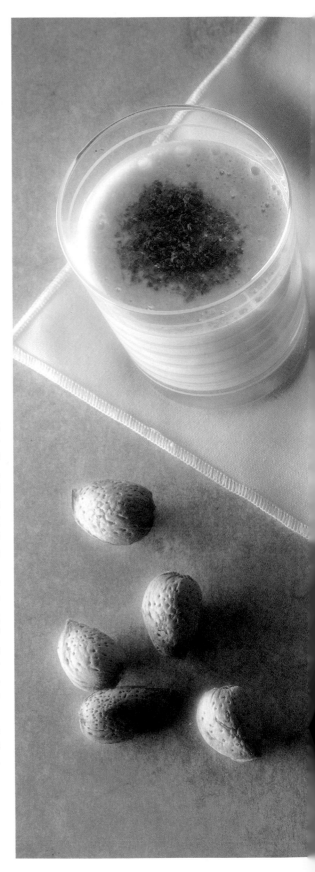

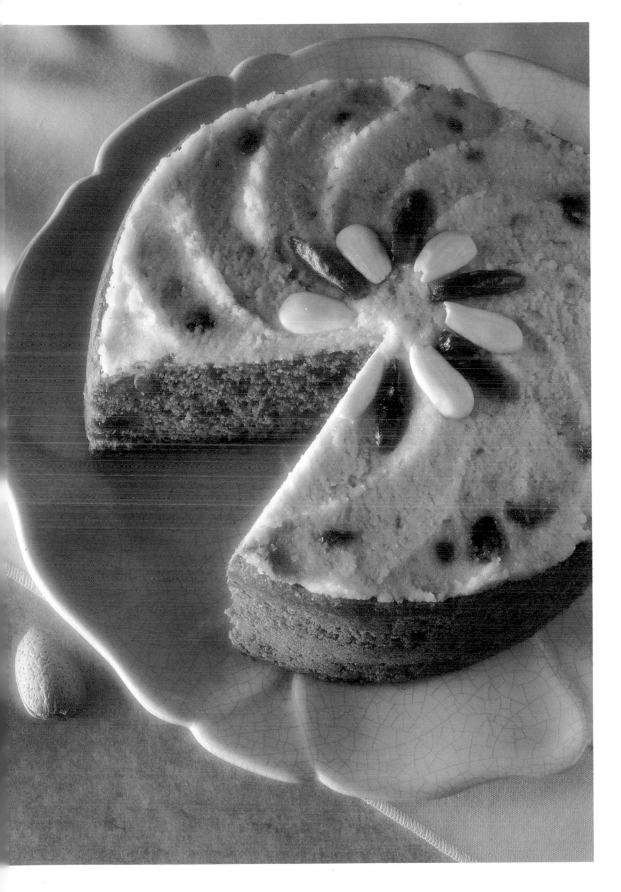

TARZAN TREAT

1 banana, peeled and cut into chunks
1 fresh peach, sliced or 100 g / 4 oz unsweetened
    peach slices
300 ml / ½ pint milk
TO DECORATE
diabetic chocolate, grated

SERVES 1
Per serving:
Energy 300 kcal / 1290 kJ
CHO   40 g (4 units)
Fibre   4 g   **Fat** 11 g   **Protein** 11 g

Place the fruit and milk into a liquidiser and blend for approximately 30 seconds, or until the fruit is thoroughly mixed into the milk. Serve in a cool tall glass topped with grated diabetic chocolate. *Illustrated on pages 104–5.*

ORANGE FIZZ

100 ml / 3½ fl oz unsweetened orange juice
200 ml / 7 fl oz sparkling mineral water
1 scoop Orange sorbet (page 68)

SERVES 1
Per serving:
Energy 62 kcal / 255 kJ
CHO   15 g (1.5 units)
Fibre   0 g   **Fat** 0 g   **Protein** 1 g

Mix together the orange juice and mineral water in a glass and top with a generous scoop of Orange sorbet. Serve the Orange fizz immediately.

STRAWBERRY YOGURT SHAKE

300 ml / ½ pint milk
75 g / 3 oz strawberries, hulled
1 strawberry yogurt

SERVES 1
Per serving:
Energy 330 kcal / 1400 kJ
CHO   40 g (4 units)
Fibre   1 g   **Fat** 12 g   **Protein** 16 g

Blend together the milk and strawberries (reserving 1 or 2 to decorate) in a liquidiser for approximately 30 seconds or until the fruit is well mixed into the milk. Slowly mix in the yogurt and pour the shake into a chilled glass. Slice the reserved strawberries and set the slices on top. Serve at once.

FOAMY APPLES

4 large dessert apples, washed and cored
1 egg
150 ml / ¼ pint unsweetened orange juice
6 drops artificial sweetener
TO DECORATE
orange slices

SERVES 4
Per serving:
Energy 80 kcal / 350 kJ
CHO   15 g (1.5 units)
Fibre   2 g   **Fat** 1 g   **Protein** 2 g

Wrap the apples in foil or in a roasting bag (pierced). Place in a roasting tin and bake in a preheated moderate oven (180°C, 350°F, Gas Mark 4) for about 40 minutes.

Meanwhile place the egg and orange juice in a bowl over a pan of hot water. Whisk for about 10 minutes until foamy and slightly thickened. Sweeten to taste. Serve on top of the unwrapped apples and decorate with the orange slices.

BANANA WHIP

2 small bananas, peeled and mashed
2 teaspooons lemon juice
artificial sweetener, if required
25 g / 1 oz almonds, finely chopped
2 teaspoons chopped stem ginger
150 g / 5 oz plain unsweetened yogurt
TO DECORATE
almonds

SERVES 2
Per serving:
Energy 200 kcal / 830 kJ
CHO 25 g (2.5 units)
Fibre 5 g **Fat** 7 g **Protein** 7 g

Place the bananas in a pan with the lemon juice. Very slowly bring the mixture to the boil and continue to cook gently for 10 minutes.

Remove the pan from the heat and allow the mixture to cool. Stir in the sweetener, almonds, ginger and yogurt. Blend well together, then spoon into two individual serving dishes. Just before serving, decorate with the almonds.

BLACKBERRY JELLY

225 g / 8 oz blackberries, washed
400 ml / 14 fl oz unsweetened apple juice
artificial sweetener (optional)
15 g / ½ oz powdered gelatine

SERVES 4
Per serving:
Energy 80 kcal / 350 kJ
CHO 15 g (1.5 units)
Fibre 4 g **Fat** 0 g **Protein** 4 g

Place the blackberries in a saucepan with the apple juice and cook gently until soft. Purée the fruit and juice in a blender. Stir in the sweetener, if used. Dissolve the gelatine in hot (not boiling) water and add to the fruit purée, then strain into a mould. Refrigerate until set. Place the mould briefly in hot water and turn out the jelly.

CREAMY ORANGE SNACK

1 wholemeal roll
1 orange, peeled, pith removed, segmented and
  chopped
50 g / 2 oz low-fat cream cheese

SERVES 1
Per serving:
Energy 260 kcal / 1120 kJ
CHO 30 g (3 units)
Fibre 4 g **Fat** 14 g **Protein** 5 g

Split the roll into two. Mix together the orange and the cream cheese, retaining one or two pieces of orange for decoration. Spread the cheese and orange mixture on to the rolls, top with the reserved orange pieces and serve.

Baking

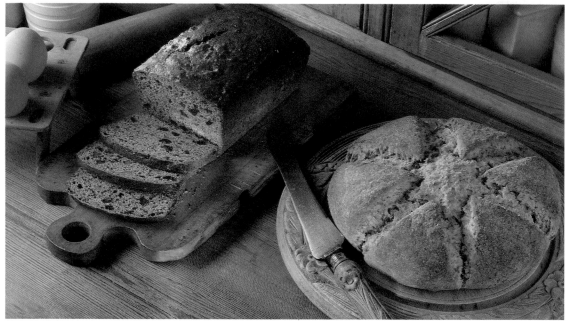

LEFT: DATE AND WALNUT BREAD; RIGHT:
BRAN LOAF

DATE AND WALNUT BREAD

225 g / 8 oz dates, stoned and chopped
50 g / 2 oz walnuts, chopped
50 g / 2 oz polyunsaturated margarine
150 ml / ¼ pint water
sugar substitute equivalent to 100 g / 4 oz caster
  sugar
1 egg
225 g / 8 oz wholemeal flour

3 teaspoons baking powder
pinch of salt

MAKES 1 × 1 kg / 2 lb loaf
Total recipe:
Energy 1990 kcal / 8365 kJ
CHO 295 g (29.5 units)
Fibre 43 g **Fat** 77 g **Protein** 46 g

Put the dates, walnuts, margarine and water into a large saucepan, bring the water just to boiling point, stir the ingredients, then remove from the heat and leave in the saucepan to cool. Add the sweetener.

Beat the egg into the date mixture. Sift the flour with the baking powder and salt. Add to the other ingredients and mix.

Spoon into a greased and floured or lined 1 kg / 2 lb loaf tin and bake in the centre of a preheated moderate oven (160°C, 325°F, Gas Mark 3) for 1¼ hours. Allow to cool in the tin for 5 minutes, then turn out.

OATMEAL BREAD

225 g / 8 oz medium oatmeal
450 ml / ¾ pint semi-skimmed milk
15 g / ½ oz fresh yeast
    or 1½ teaspoons dried yeast with 1 teaspoon
    sugar
4 tablespoons warm water
2–3 teaspoons salt
50 g / 2 oz polyunsaturated margarine, melted
225 g / 8 oz strong white or unbleached flour

TO FINISH
milk
coarse oatmeal

MAKES 1 small loaf
Total recipe:
Energy 2245 kcal / 9475 kJ
CHO 350 g (35 units)
Fibre 22 g **Fat** 71 g **Protein** 68 g

Put the oatmeal into a mixing bowl and add the milk. Leave to soak overnight for the oatmeal to absorb the milk.

Dissolve the yeast in the warm water, adding the sugar if using dried yeast, and leave for 10 minutes to froth. Mix the yeast liquid into the oatmeal which will be of porridge consistency, with the salt and melted margarine.

Sift and beat in sufficient white flour to make a smooth, very soft dough. Knead thoroughly on a thickly floured board, adding more flour if necessary. (A dough hook on a mixer at lowest speed will cut the kneading time to about 5 minutes.) Replace in a warm bowl, cover with a damp cloth and leave in a warm place to rise for 1½–2 hours or until the dough has doubled in bulk.

Knock back the dough on a board sprinkled with medium oatmeal. Divide in two and put one half into a warmed and greased 450 g / 1 lb loaf tin. It should half-fill the tin. Cover and prove for about 45 minutes or until the dough rises to the top of the tin.

Brush with milk and sprinkle with coarse oatmeal. Bake in a preheated hot oven (220°C, 425°F, Gas Mark 7) for 20–30 minutes. Lower the heat to 160°C, 325°F, Gas Mark 3 and bake for a further 15–20 minutes. Remove from the tin and tap the bottom to see if it sounds hollow. Cool on a wire tray.

BRAN LOAF

350 g / 12 oz self-raising flour
½ teaspoon salt
100 g / 4 oz polyunsaturated margarine
25 g / 1 oz bran
200 ml / ⅓ pint semi-skimmed milk

MAKES 1 × 18 cm / 7 inch round loaf
Total recipe:
Energy 2075 kcal / 8120 kJ
CHO 290 g (29 units)
Fibre 23 g **Fat** 90 g **Protein** 43 g

If using plain or wholewheat flour in place of self-raising, add 3 tablespoons baking powder.

Sift the flour with the salt. Rub in the margarine until the mixture is like fine breadcrumbs. Add the bran and milk. Knead the mixture and roll out to an 18 cm / 7 inch round. Place on a well-greased baking sheet and mark into 6–8 portions. Bake in the centre of a preheated moderately hot oven (200°C, 400°F, Gas Mark 6) for 30–35 minutes.

SOFT WHOLEMEAL ROLLS

225 g/8 oz wholemeal flour
1 teaspoon salt
25 g/1 oz polyunsaturated margarine
15 g/½ oz fresh yeast
150 ml/¼ pint (approximately) tepid milk

MAKES 8 rolls
Per roll:
Energy 125 kcal/525 kJ
CHO 20 g (2 units)
Fibre 2 g   **Fat** 3 g   **Protein** 4 g

Sift the flour with the salt into a mixing bowl and warm. Rub in the fat. Blend the fresh yeast with the tepid milk and leave for 10 minutes to froth.

Pour the yeast liquid into the flour and mix, adding a little more milk if necessary. Beat until the dough leaves the sides of the bowl clean, turn on to a floured board and knead for 10 minutes. Put the dough into an oiled polythene bag and leave to rise until doubled in bulk.

Knock back the dough, make a fat sausage shape and cut across into eight equal-sized pieces. Shape into rounds or ovals. Press down firmly with the heel of your hand and release. Place on a floured baking sheet, leaving space between them for expansion. Cover and prove for 15 minutes or until doubled in size.

Dust with flour and bake in the centre of a preheated very hot oven (230°C, 450°F, Gas Mark 8) for 15–20 minutes. When cooked, remove to a wire tray and cover with a teatowel.

MUSHROOM BREAD

25 g/1 oz fresh yeast
150 ml/¼ pint warm water
750 g/1½–1¾ lb wholemeal flour
350 g/12 oz plain flour
1 tablespoon salt
25 g/1 oz bran
25 g/1 oz polyunsaturated margarine
150 ml/¼ pint semi-skimmed milk

25 g/1 oz onion, finely chopped
225 g/8 oz mushrooms, chopped

MAKES 2 × 1 kg/2 lb loaves
Total recipe:
Energy 3930 kcal/16665 kJ
CHO 770 g (77 units)
Fibre 99 g   **Fat** 47 g   **Protein** 151 g

Blend the yeast with 3 tablespoons of the water and leave for 10 minutes to froth.

Sift the flours and salt into a warmed bowl. Add the bran and rub in the margarine. Make a well in the centre and pour in the yeast liquid with the remaining water and milk. Draw all the ingredients together and beat until the dough is smooth and comes cleanly away from the sides of the bowl. Turn out on to a floured surface and knead for 5–8 minutes or until smooth and elastic. Place in a greased bowl, cover with a damp cloth and leave in a warm place to rise until it has doubled its bulk.

Turn out on to a floured surface and knead in the onion and mushrooms a little at a time, using a little extra flour should the dough become too sticky. Knead for 2 minutes, then divide the mixture in half and shape into two loaves. Place in two greased 1 kg/2 lb loaf tins, leave in a warm place and prove until the dough reaches the top of the tins.

Bake in a preheated hot oven (220°C, 425°F, Gas Mark 7) for 20 minutes, then reduce the heat to 190°C, 375°F, Gas Mark 5 and bake for a further 30 minutes until the bread sounds hollow when tapped underneath. Cool on a wire tray.

YOGURT AND BANANA LOAF

1 teaspoon dried yeast
2 tablespoons warm water
2 ripe bananas, peeled
50 g/2 oz polyunsaturated margarine
120 ml/4 fl oz plain unsweetened yogurt
1 egg
150 g/5 oz wholemeal flour
150 g/5 oz strong white flour
½ teaspoon salt
1 tablespoon grated lemon rind

1 tablespoon grated orange rind
50 g/2 oz walnuts, chopped
25 g/1 oz raisins

MAKES 1 × 1 kg/2 lb loaf
Total recipe:
Energy 1970 kcal/8280 kJ
CHO 275 g (27.5 units)
Fibre 30 g **Fat** 80 g **Protein** 56 g

Dissolve the yeast in the warm water and leave for 10 minutes to froth. Blend or mash together the bananas, margarine, yogurt and egg. Add the yeast mixture.

Blend the flours, keeping 100 g/4 oz of the wholemeal flour in reserve, salt, orange and lemon rinds. Stir in the banana and yeast mixture. Cover and leave to rise in a warm place for 1 hour.

Fold in the walnuts, raisins and remaining wholemeal flour and put into a greased, floured 1 kg/2 lb bread tin. Cover and allow to rise for a further 30 minutes.

Bake in a preheated moderate oven (180°C, 350°F, Gas Mark 4) for 70 minutes. Allow to become quite cold before slicing.

APRICOT AND WALNUT LOAF

225 g/8 oz wholemeal flour
225 g/8 oz strong white flour
100 g/4 oz dried apricots, snipped
50 g/2 oz walnuts, chopped
15 g/1½ oz fresh yeast, or 1½ teaspoons dried
    yeast with 1 teaspoon sugar
300 ml/1½ pint tepid milk and water
50 g/2 oz polyunsaturated margarine, cut up
1 egg, beaten

MAKES 2 × 450 g/1 lb loaves
Total recipe:
Energy 2470 kcal/10395 kJ
CHO 370 g (37 units)
Fibre 54 g **Fat** 85 g **Protein** 77 g

Sift the flours into a warm mixing bowl. Mix in the apricots and walnuts.

Dissolve the yeast in half the milk and water, adding the sugar if using dried yeast. Leave for 10 minutes or until frothy.

Melt the margarine in the remaining milk and water. Stir in the beaten egg. Add all the liquids to the dry ingredients and mix to a smooth dough. Knead well, cover and put into a warm place to rise until doubled in bulk.

Turn on to a floured board, knock back the dough and divide in half. Put into two warmed and greased 450 g/1 lb loaf tins. Cover and prove in a warm place until the dough fills the tins.

Bake in a preheated very hot oven (230°C, 450°F, Gas Mark 8) for 20 minutes. Reduce the heat to 200°C, 400°C, Gas Mark 6 and cook for a further 15–20 minutes. Allow to shrink slightly, unmould and cool on a wire tray.

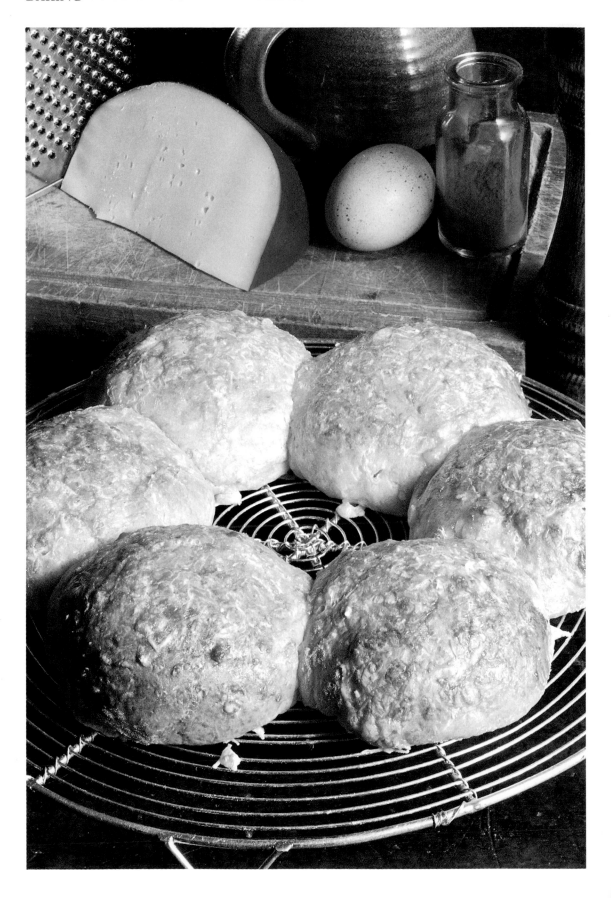

SPICED CARROT LOAF

225 g/8 oz wholemeal flour
225 g/8 oz strong white flour
1 teaspoon dried yeast
150 ml/¼ pint tepid water
100 g/4 oz grated carrot
2 eggs, beaten
75 g/3 oz polyunsaturated margarine, melted
2 teaspoons grated orange rind
1 teaspoon cinnamon

1 teaspoon mixed spice
½ teaspoon salt

MAKES 1 × 450 g/1 lb loaf
Total recipe:
Energy 2215 kcal/9330 kJ
CHO 320 g (32 units)
Fibre 31 g **Fat** 81 g **Protein** 70 g

Sift the flours together in a bowl. Dissolve the yeast in the water in a mixing bowl. Add the grated carrot, beaten eggs and half the flour. Mix well, cover with a cloth and leave in a warm place to rise for 1 hour. Add the remaining flour, melted margarine, orange rind, spices and salt. Knead, then cover and leave in a warm place to rise for a further 30 minutes.

Place the risen dough in a greased, floured 450 g/1 lb loaf tin, cover and leave to rise for a further 15 minutes. Bake in a preheated moderately hot oven (190°C, 375°F, Gas Mark 5) for 45 minutes. Remove from the tin and cool before slicing.

EDAM TEA RING

225 g/8 oz plain flour
4½ teaspoons baking powder
1 teaspoon salt
1 teaspoon paprika
225 g/8 oz Edam cheese, grated
4 tablespoons piccalilli pickle, chopped
1 large egg
150 ml/¼ pint semi-skimmed milk

SERVES 6
Per serving:
Energy 270 kcal/1130 kJ
CHO 26 g (2.5 units)
Fibre 2 g **Fat** 11 g **Protein** 16 g

Sift the flour, baking powder, salt and paprika pepper into a large mixing bowl. Rub in 200 g/7 oz of the grated cheese and add the piccalilli pickle.

Beat the egg and milk together. Pour most of the milk mixture into the cheese mixture, reserving a little for glazing.

Divide the dough into six pieces, and form each into a roll. Place these on a baking sheet to form a circle, leaving a space between each roll. Brush the rolls with the milk and egg mixture and sprinkle with the remaining cheese. Bake in a preheated hot oven (220°C, 425°F, Gas Mark 7) for 25 minutes. Cool on a wire tray. Serve as a circle, or broken up, either hot or cold.

RICH BRAN SCONES

200 g / 7 oz wholemeal flour
1 teaspoon baking powder
25 g / 1 oz bran
salt
50 g / 2 oz polyunsaturated margarine
2 tablespoons currants or sultanas
1 egg, mixed with milk to make up to 150 ml /
*   ¼ pint*
milk for glazing

TO DECORATE
sesame seeds

MAKES 10 scones
Per scone:
Energy 130 kcal / 550 kJ
CHO   15 g (1.5 units)
Fibre   3 g   **Fat** 5 g   **Protein** 4 g

Mix the flour, baking powder, bran and salt in a bowl and rub in the margarine. Stir in the fruit. Beat the egg and milk together and add to the flour mixture to make a soft dough.

Turn on to a floured surface. Roll out to 1 cm / ½ inch thickness and cut into rounds with a 6 cm / 2½ inch diameter cutter. Place the scones on a greased baking sheet, brush the tops with milk and sprinkle with sesame seeds. Bake in a preheated hot oven (220°C, 425°F, Gas Mark 7) for 10–12 minutes or until golden.

HERB SCONES

250 ml / 8 fl oz water
65 g / 2½ oz polyunsaturated margarine
175 g / 6 oz wholemeal flour
3 eggs
275 g / 10 oz freshly mashed potatoes
salt and freshly ground black pepper
4 tablespoons chopped mixed herbs (chervil,
*   dill, chives and parsley)*

MAKES 16 scones
Per scone:
Energy 90 kcal / 400 kJ
CHO   10 g (1 unit)
Fibre   1 g   **Fat** 4 g   **Protein** 3 g

Boil the water and margarine together in a large saucepan. When the margarine has melted, remove from the heat and add the flour. Stir until it forms a thick paste. Break in the eggs, one at a time, and continue to beat until the mixture is smooth and comes away from the sides of the pan. Beat in the hot mashed potatoes and continue beating until they are amalgamated. Add salt and pepper to taste. Stir in the chopped herbs. Leave to cool.

Heat a lightly greased griddle until very hot, then form the mixture into flat round cakes and cook them until golden brown, turning once. Serve hot.

WHOLEMEAL PASTRY

225 g / 8 oz wholemeal flour
pinch of salt
100 g / 4 oz polyunsaturated margarine
2 egg yolks
1 tablespoon cold water

MAKES 225 g / 8 oz pastry
Total recipe:
Energy 1650 kcal / 6880 kJ
CHO   150 g (15 units)
Fibre   21 g   **Fat** 103 g   **Protein** 39 g

As this pastry is a little difficult to handle, it is best to roll it out on a piece of foil so that it can be easily lifted.

Put the flour and salt in a bowl, then rub in the margarine until the mixture resembles fine breadcrumbs. Beat the egg yolks with the water, then add to the dry mixture and mix to a dough.

HERB BISCUITS

50 g/2 oz wholemeal flour
25 g/1 oz polyunsaturated margarine
pinch of salt
pinch of cayenne
50 g/2 oz Cheddar cheese, grated
½ teaspoon caraway seeds or dried dill seeds
½ teaspoon Dijon mustard
1 egg yolk, lightly beaten
1 tablespoon iced water

MAKES 20 biscuits
Per biscuit:
Energy 30 kcal/130 kJ
CHO 0 g (0 units)
Fibre 0 g **Fat** 2 g **Protein** 1 g

Sift the flour into a bowl and rub in the margarine in small pieces. Add the salt and cayenne and mix in the grated cheese with the blade of a knife. (Alternatively, all this can be done in a mixer or food processor.) Stir in the caraway seeds (or dill). Stir the mustard into the egg yolk and stir into the mixture. Add enough of the iced water to give a soft but firm dough. Wrap loosely in cling film and chill for 1 hour in the refrigerator.

Roll out on a floured board until about 3 mm/⅛ inch thick and cut into small rounds. Lay the biscuits on a greased baking sheet and bake in a preheated moderately hot oven (200°C, 400°F, Gas Mark 6) for 7 minutes or until golden brown and puffed up. Serve immediately.

HERBED BREAD ROUND

225 g/8 oz plain flour
225 g/8 oz wholemeal flour
½ teaspoon salt
1 teaspoon bicarbonate of soda
25 g/1 oz polyunsaturated margarine
2 large onions, grated
3 celery sticks, sliced
1 teaspoon dried mixed herbs
2 tablespoons chopped parsley

250 ml/8 fl oz plain unsweetened yogurt
little milk to glaze

SERVES 8
Per serving:
Energy 230 kcal/980 kJ
CHO 40 g (4 units)
Fibre 4 g **Fat** 3 g **Protein** 8 g

Combine the flours, salt and soda in a large mixing bowl. Rub in the margarine, then stir in the onions, celery and herbs. Mix well. Add enough of the yogurt to give a soft dough. Turn out on to a lightly floured surface and knead lightly. Shape into a 22 cm/9 inch round and place on a baking sheet. Score the top into eight sections and glaze with a little milk. Bake in a preheated moderately hot oven (200°C, 400°F, Gas Mark 6) for 30–35 minutes, until well risen and golden.

Snacks

TUNA AND PEPPER OMELETTES

1 green pepper, cored, seeded and sliced
1 × 200 g/7 oz can tuna fish, drained and
   flaked
100 g/4 oz cooked peas
2 tomatoes, skinned and chopped
salt
freshly ground black pepper
OMELETTE MIXTURE
8 eggs
2 tablespoons water
salt

freshly ground black pepper
25 g/1 oz polyunsaturated margarine
TO GARNISH
tomato slices
chopped parsley

SERVES 4
Per serving:
Energy 380 kcal/1600 kJ
CHO 0 g (0 units)
Fibre 3 g   **Fat** 28 g   **Protein** 27 g

Cook the green pepper in boiling water for 2–3 minutes, then drain. Place in a saucepan and add the remaining ingredients, with salt and pepper to taste. Heat through gently while making the omelettes.

Beat the eggs with the water and salt and pepper to taste. Melt a quarter of the margarine in an omelette pan and pour in a quarter of the egg mixture. Cook over a moderate heat, moving the cooked mixture towards the centre with a palette knife. When the omelette is just cooked, place a quarter of the filling on one side and fold over. Transfer to a warmed serving plate and keep warm while making three more omelettes with the remaining ingredients. Garnish with tomato slices and parsley. Serve immediately.

OVEN POTATO OMELETTE

25 g/1 oz polyunsaturated margarine
2 large cooked potatoes, sliced
2 canned red peppers, cut into small pieces
6–8 eggs
2 tablespoons milk
salt
freshly ground black pepper
1 tablespoon chopped chives

1 tablespoon chopped parsley
1 teaspoon grated lemon rind

SERVES 4
Per serving:
Energy 240 kcal/1000 kJ
CHO 10 g (1 unit)
Fibre 1 g   **Fat** 16 g   **Protein** 13 g

Put the margarine into a 20–23 cm (8–9 inch) round ovenproof dish and heat towards the top of a preheated hot oven (220°C, 425°F, Gas Mark 7) until melted. Add the potatoes and peppers and heat for another few minutes. Beat the eggs with the remaining ingredients, pour over the potato and pepper mixture, return to the oven, just above the centre. Bake for 10–15 minutes or until set to personal taste.

RICE BALLS IN TOMATO SAUCE

225 g/8 oz brown rice
1 egg, lightly beaten
1 tablespoon wholemeal flour
100 g/4 oz Mozzarella cheese, cubed
SAUCE
25 g/1 oz polyunsaturated margarine
1 large onion (about 350 g/12 oz), finely
  chopped
500 g/1¼ lb tomatoes, skinned, seeded and
  chopped or 1 × 400 g (14 oz) can tomatoes,
  drained and chopped
1 teaspoon dried basil

½ teaspoon dried thyme
salt
freshly ground black pepper
300 ml/½ pint light stock
TO GARNISH
1 tablespoon finely chopped parsley

SERVES 4
Per serving:
Energy 370 kcal/1570 kJ
CHO 55 g (5.5 units)
Fibre 5 g **Fat** 13 g **Protein** 11 g

To make the sauce, melt the margarine in a saucepan. Add the onion and fry for 5 minutes or until soft. Add the tomatoes, basil, thyme, salt and pepper and cook for a further 3 minutes. Stir in the stock. Bring to the boil, then simmer, covered, for 15 minutes.

Meanwhile, cook the rice in boiling salted water for 15 minutes or until tender. Drain well and allow to cool. Mix the rice with the egg and flour. Take a large spoonful of the rice mixture, roll into a ball and insert a cube of cheese. Completely enclose the cube of cheese. Continue making the rice balls until all the rice mixture and cheese have been used.

Add the rice balls to the sauce and simmer for a further 10 minutes.

To serve, turn the rice balls and the sauce into a warmed serving dish and sprinkle with the parsley.

HAM AND PINEAPPLE KEBABS

75–100 g/3–4 oz fresh coconut
175 g/6 oz brown rice
350 ml/12 fl oz water
salt
KEBABS
½ large or 1 small pineapple, peeled and cut
  into 2 cm/1¾ inch cubes
450 g/1 lb cooked ham, cut in 1 thick slice and
  diced
1 tablespoon polyunsaturated vegetable oil

¼ teaspoon ground ginger
SAUCE
300 ml/½ pint plain unsweetened yogurt
1–2 teaspoons curry powder

SERVES 4
Per serving:
Energy 450 kcal/1875 kJ
CHO 50 g (5 units)
Fibre 5 g **Fat** 15 g **Protein** 28 g

Rub the coconut against the coarse side of a grater, put into a saucepan and heat very gently until lightly browned. Remove half of the coconut from the saucepan, put on one side. Add the rice, water and a pinch of salt to the coconut in the saucepan. Bring the water to the boil. Stir briskly with a fork, cover the pan, lower the heat and simmer for 15 minutes.

Meanwhile, thread the pineapple and ham on to metal skewers. Blend the oil and ginger; brush over the pineapple and ham. Cook the kebabs under a preheated grill for 2–3 minutes.

To make the sauce, blend the yogurt and curry paste. Spoon into a sauceboat.

Serve the coconut rice on a heated dish, and place the kebabs on top. Sprinkle with the remaining coconut.

FILLED PITTA BREAD

1 wholemeal pitta bread
1 teaspoon polyunsaturated margarine
25 g/1 oz French beans, cooked and chopped
50 g/2 oz tuna fish, drained and chopped
25 g/1 oz red pepper, chopped
25 g/1 oz green pepper, chopped
4 black olives, stoned
salt and freshly ground black pepper

SERVES 1
Per serving:
Energy 430 kcal/1820 kJ
CHO 45 g (4.5 units)
Fibre 6 g   **Fat** 19 g   **Protein** 19 g

Slit the pitta bread down one side and spread the inside with the margarine. Mix the remaining ingredients together with salt and pepper to taste and spoon into the bread. Serve immediately.

FILLED PITTA BREAD

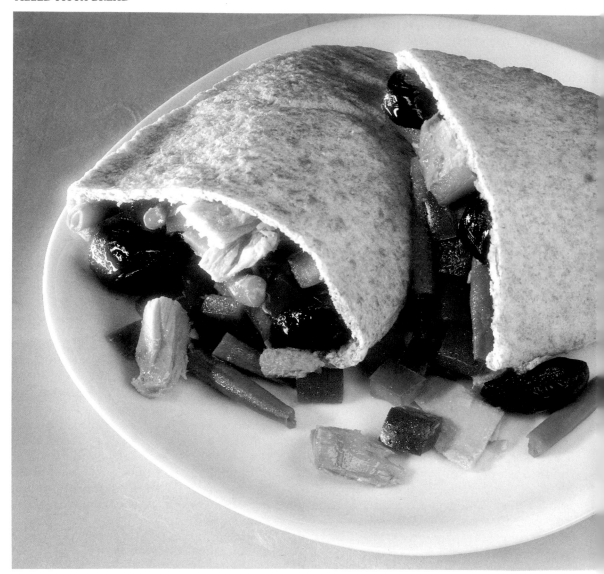

BARBECUE BUTTER BEANS

1 tablespoon polyunsaturated vegetable oil
1 onion, chopped
1 garlic clove, crushed
2 tomatoes, skinned
drop of artificial sweetener
pinch of dry mustard
pinch of chilli powder
1 tablespoon tomato purée
1 × 275 g (10 oz) can butter beans, drained

SERVES 4
Per serving:
Energy 90 kcal / 380 kJ
CHO 10 g (1 unit)
Fibre 3 g   **Fat** 2 g   **Protein** 5 g

Heat the oil in a saucepan, add the onion and garlic and cook until softened. Add the remaining ingredients, except the beans, and simmer for 10 minutes. Stir in the beans, heat thoroughly and serve.

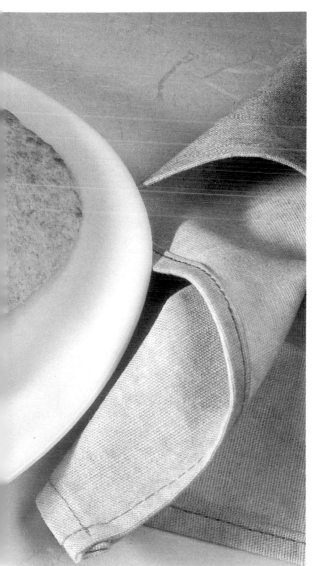

TUNA-STUFFED TOMATOES

1 × 200 g (7 oz) can tuna fish, drained and
  flaked
1 medium celery stick, chopped
2 tablespoons finely chopped onion
2 tablespoons finely chopped green pepper
3 tablespoons lemon juice
freshly ground black pepper
4 large tomatoes
salt
6 lettuce leaves
TO GARNISH
4 lemon slices, twisted

SERVES 4
Per serving:
Energy 160 kcal / 660 kJ
CHO 0 g (0 units)
Fibre 1 g   **Fat** 11 g   **Protein** 12 g

Mix together the tuna, celery, onion, green pepper, lemon juice and pepper to taste. Chill the mixture.

With stem end down, cut each tomato into six wedges, cutting down to, but not through, the base. Spread the wedges apart slightly and sprinkle lightly with salt. Place the lettuce leaves on a serving plate. Arrange the tomatoes on the lettuce. Spoon equal amounts of the tuna mixture into the centre of each tomato. Garnish with twists of lemon and serve.

CHICKEN TOASTIES

100 g/4 oz cold cooked chicken, diced
100 g/4 oz cooked sweetcorn
6 tablespoons plain unsweetened yogurt

8 slices wholemeal bread
25 g/1 oz polyunsaturated margarine

SERVES 2–4

2 servings			4 servings		
Per serving:			**Per serving:**		
Energy 515 kcal/2180 kJ			**Energy** 345 kcal/1450 kJ		
CHO 65 g (6.5 units)			**CHO** 40 g (4 units)		
Fibre 13 g	**Fat** 16 g	**Protein** 30 g	**Fibre** 8 g	**Fat** 11 g	**Protein** 20 g

Combine the chicken, sweetcorn and yogurt. Spread the bread with the margarine and trim to fit a sandwich toaster. Place the bread 'sunnyside down' in the toaster and spoon some of the filling into the centre. Place another slice of bread 'sunnyside up' on top and cook according to the toaster manufacturer's instructions.

HOT CHILLI FISH CURRY

15 g/½ oz polyunsaturated margarine
1 tablespoon curry powder
1 teaspoon chilli powder
2 onions, chopped
1 garlic clove, crushed
600 ml/1 pint chicken stock
2 tablespoons tomato purée
3 tablespoons lemon juice
salt

450 g/1 lb cooked white fish fillets, diced, or
225 g/8 oz peeled prawns

SERVES 4

Per serving:		
Energy 100 kcal/445 kJ		
CHO 5 g (0.5 units)		
Fibre 0 g	**Fat** 4 g	**Protein** 13 g

Melt the margarine in a saucepan, add the curry and chilli powders and cook over a low heat for 1 minute. Add the onions and garlic and fry for 3 minutes. Stir in the stock, tomato purée and lemon juice. Cover and simmer for 1 hour. The sauce should be quite thick.

Stir in the fish and cook for a further 10 minutes; if using prawns, cook for 5 minutes only. Taste and add salt if required. Serve with rice.

WHOLEMEAL MACARONI CARBONARA

350–450 g/12 oz–1 lb wholemeal macaroni
15 g/½ oz polyunsaturated margarine
175 g/6 oz cooked ham, cut into short thin strips
salt
freshly ground black pepper
2 tablespoons milk
3 eggs
about 50 g/2 oz grated Parmesan cheese

SERVES 6

Per serving:		
Energy 350 kcal/1480 kJ		
CHO 45 g (4.5 units)		
Fibre 0 g	**Fat** 10 g	**Protein** 12 g

Cook the macaroni in boiling water for 10–15 minutes or until tender.

Meanwhile, melt the margarine in a large pan, add the ham and fry gently until it is fairly crisp. Add a little salt, depending upon how salty the ham is, and plenty of pepper.

In a bowl beat the milk with the eggs.

Drain the macaroni and stir into the ham. Turn off the heat and add the beaten egg mixture, stirring constantly. The eggs will cook and thicken slightly from the warmth of the pasta. Serve at once on hot plates and sprinkle with Parmesan cheese. A tomato salad makes an interesting and colourful accompaniment.

SPAGHETTI WITH ALMOND CHEESE

350 g/12 oz wholemeal spaghetti
salt
1 tablespoon chopped parsley
freshly ground black pepper
SAUCE
25 g/1 oz grated Parmesan cheese
100 g/4 oz ground almonds
100 g/4 oz cottage cheese
pinch of grated nutmeg
pinch of grated cinnamon

3 tablespoons plain unsweetened yogurt
150 ml/¼ pint liquid from cooking spaghetti
TO GARNISH
25 g/1 oz browned flaked almonds

SERVES 4
Per serving:
Energy 400 kcal/1670 kJ
CHO 50 g (5 units)
Fibre 2 g **Fat** 14 g **Protein** 17 g

Cook the spaghetti for 10–15 minutes in boiling salted water. Drain, saving 150 ml/¼ pint of the water for the sauce and mix the spaghetti with the parsley and pepper to taste. Put the spaghetti in a large heated dish and keep hot.

Mix together all the sauce ingredients and season well with salt and pepper. Spoon over the spaghetti and garnish with the almonds.

CHEESE POTS

1 celery stick, diced
1 large ripe dessert pear, peeled, cored and diced
1 large dessert apple, peeled, cored and diced
½–1 teaspoon chopped chives
½–1 tablespoon lemon juice
225 g/8 oz Lancashire or crumbly Cheddar cheese
TO GARNISH
1 tablespoon chopped parsley
paprika

SERVES 4
Per serving:
Energy 260 kcal/1090 kJ
CHO 10 g (1 unit)
Fibre 1 g **Fat** 18 g **Protein** 15 g

Toss the celery, pear and apple dice with the chives and lemon juice.

Divide the mixture between four individual flameproof or ovenproof dishes. You should use flameproof dishes if heating under the grill. Crumble the cheese over the fruit and celery. Place under a preheated grill for 5–6 minutes or until golden brown on top or towards the top of a preheated hot oven (220°C, 425°F, Gas Mark 7) for 10 minutes.

Garnish with the parsley and a sprinkling of paprika.

TUNA AND GRAPEFRUIT CAKE

*1 × 200 g (7 oz) can tuna fish, drained and
    flaked*
1 tablespoon grated grapefruit rind
2–3 tablespoons grapefruit juice
25 g/1 oz dried milk powder

4 tablespoons cold water
50 g/2 oz fresh breadcrumbs
1 egg, beaten
1 small onion, grated
½ teaspoon paprika

SERVES 4–6

4 servings			**6 servings**		
Per serving:			**Per serving:**		
Energy 160 kcal/685 kJ			**Energy** 135 kcal/570 kJ		
CHO 5 g (0.5 units)			**CHO** 5 g (0.5 units)		
Fibre 1 g	**Fat** 10 g	**Protein** 11 g	**Fibre** 0 g	**Fat** 8 g	**Protein** 9 g

Mix the tuna with the grapefruit rind and
juice. Dissolve the milk powder in the
water and add to the tuna with the remaining
ingredients. Mix well.

Spoon into a lightly greased 450 ml (¾
pint) shallow baking dish and smooth the
top. Bake in a preheated moderate oven
(180°C, 350°F, Gas Mark 4) for 40 minutes
or until set and golden brown. Cool slightly
in the dish, then turn out on to a serving
plate and leave to cool completely. Serve
cold, cut into slices.

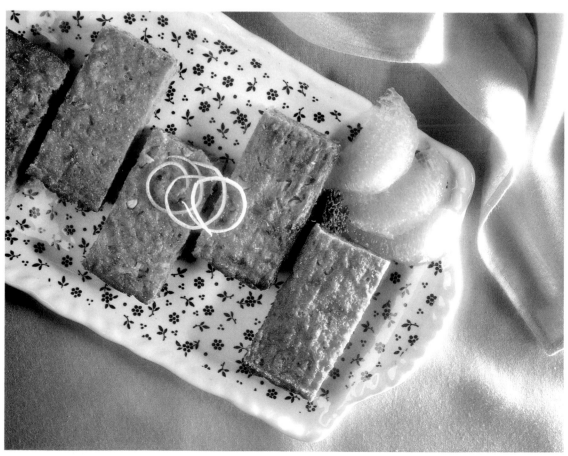

TUNA AND GRAPEFRUIT CAKE

MEAL PLANS

The following menus show how recipes from this book may be combined to provide well-balanced daily eating plans. The plans are calculated at varying energy levels, from 1000 kcal/4200 kJ a day up to 2500 kcal/10000 kJ, the lower levels being suitable for inclusion in weight-reducing diets, and the two upper levels providing guidelines for women and men respectively whose weights are satisfactory; very active people may require a higher energy intake to maintain their ideal weight.

1000 kcal/4200 kJ

PLAN 1
300 ml/½ pint skimmed milk

BREAKFAST
30 g/1½ oz Storecupboard muesli
200 ml/⅓ pint unsweetened fruit juice
MID MORNING
tea or coffee
LUNCH
Horenso Tamagi Maki
1 slice wholemeal bread
scrape polyunsaturated margarine
fresh fruit
MID AFTERNOON
tea or coffee
EVENING MEAL
Dolmas
50 g/2 oz brown rice
Orange surprise
BEDTIME
tea or coffee

PLAN 2
300 ml/½ pint skimmed milk

BREAKFAST
Orange and prune crunch
200 ml/⅓ pint fruit juice, unsweetened
MID MORNING
tea or coffee
LUNCH
Broad bean and ham salad
1 slice wholemeal bread
scrape polyunsaturated margarine
apple
MID AFTERNOON
tea or coffee
EVENING MEAL
Chicken bake with yogurt topping
green beans
2 boiled new potatoes
Grapes and oranges
BEDTIME
tea or coffee

1500 kcal/6300 kJ

PLAN 1
300 ml/½ pint skimmed milk

BREAKFAST
2 slices wholemeal bread
scrape polyunsaturated margarine
grilled mushrooms and tomatoes

PLAN 2
300 ml/½ pint skimmed milk

BREAKFAST
1 helping (half recipe) Yogurt and oat
   muesli
200 ml/⅓ pint fruit juice, unsweetened

MID MORNING
tea or coffee
LUNCH
Wholemeal macaroni carbonara
fresh fruit
MID AFTERNOON
tea or coffee
EVENING MEAL
Lentil soup with coconut
Smoked cod jumble
green beans
Apricot soufflé
BEDTIME
2 Soft wholemeal rolls
tea or coffee

MID MORNING
tea or coffee
LUNCH
Napoleon's bean salad
2 slices wholemeal bread
scrape polyunsaturated margarine
pear
MID AFTERNOON
tea or coffee
EVENING MEAL
Gazpacho
Black-eye pea casserole
salad
Grape-stuffed apples
BEDTIME
tea or coffee
1 Rich bran scone
scrape polyunsaturated margarine

2000 kcal/8400 kJ

PLAN 1
600 ml/1 pint skimmed milk

BREAKFAST
Yogurt and oat muesli
1 slice wholemeal bread
scrape polyunsaturated margarine
200 ml/⅓ pint unsweetened fruit juice
MID MORNING
tea or coffee
1 Rich bran scone
scrape polyunsaturated margarine
LUNCH
Barbecue butter beans
jacket potato
Rhubarb and ginger soufflé
MID AFTERNOON
tea or coffee
EVENING MEAL
Vegetable soup
Leek pie
carrots and peas
Grape jelly
BEDTIME
tea or coffee
1 slice Yogurt and banana loaf

PLAN 2
600 ml/1 pint skimmed milk

BREAKFAST
Breakfast scramble
2 slices wholemeal bread
scrape polyunsaturated margarine
MID MORNING
tea or coffee
2 Soft wholemeal rolls
LUNCH
Potato and tomato pie
salad
Banana whip
MID AFTERNOON
tea or coffee
fresh fruit
EVENING MEAL
Spicy vegetable curry
50 g/2 oz brown rice, boiled
Lemon and blackcurrant dessert
BEDTIME
tea or coffee
2 Rich bran scones
scrape polyunsaturated margarine

2500 kcal/10500 kJ

PLAN 1
600 ml/1 pint skimmed milk

BREAKFAST
Breakfast scramble
2 slices wholemeal bread
scrape polyunsaturated margarine
200 ml/⅓ pint unsweetened fruit juice
MID MORNING
tea or coffee
1 slice Apricot and walnut loaf
LUNCH
Filled pitta bread
side salad
Orange sorbet
MID AFTERNOON
tea or coffee
2 Rich bran scones
scrape polyunsaturated margarine
EVENING MEAL
Tuna fish pâté
Curried chicken with coriander
50 g/2 oz brown rice
Peach and raspberry cheesecake
BEDTIME
tea or coffee
1 slice Chocolate cake

PLAN 2
600 ml/1 pint skimmed milk

BREAKFAST
Brown rice piperade
grilled tomato
200 ml/⅓ pint fruit juice, unsweetened
MID MORNING
tea or coffee
1 section Herbed bread round
scrape polyunsaturated margarine
LUNCH
Ham and pineapple kebabs
Rhubarb fool
MID AFTERNOON
tea or coffee
1 Soft wholemeal roll
scrape polyunsaturated margarine
EVENING MEAL
Gardeners' broth
Winter casserole
Ratatouille
Bramble mousse
BEDTIME
tea or coffee
Edam tea ring

INDEX

Page numbers in italics indicate
illustrations